PARKINSON'S DISEASE

The Complete Guide for Patients and Caregivers

ABRAHAM N. LIEBERMAN, M.D.
Chief of Movement Disorders, Barrow Neurological Institute
FRANK L. WILLIAMS
Executive Director, American Parkinson's Disease Association
SUSAN IMKE, R.N., M.S.
ELLEN MOSCINSKI, L.C.S.W., M.S.W.
PAULA BENOIST FALWELL, P.T.
HARLEY GORDON, ESQ.

with SUZANNE LEVERT

Produced by
THE PHILIP LIEF GROUP, INC.

A FIRESIDE BOOK
Published by Simon & Schuster
New York   *London*   *Toronto*   *Sydney*   *Tokyo*   *Singapore*

FIRESIDE
Simon & Schuster Building
Rockefeller Center
1230 Avenue of the Americas
New York, New York 10020

Designed by Irving Perkins Associates

Manufactured in the United States of America

3   5   7   9   10   8   6   4   2

Library of Congress Cataloging-in-Publication Data

Parkinson's disease: the complete guide for patients and caregivers /
Abraham N. Lieberman . . . [et al.].
        p.   cm.
"Produced by the Philip Lief Group, Inc."
"A Fireside book."
Includes index.
1. Parkinsonism—Popular works.   I. Lieberman, A. (Abraham), date.
RC382.P325   1993
616.8'33—dc20
92-21419
CIP

ISBN 0-671-76819-0

Produced by The Philip Lief Group, Inc.
6 West 20th Street
New York, New York 10011

Grateful acknowledgment is made to the following for permission to reprint material: chart of contraindicated drugs, courtesy of the Milwaukee Chapter of the APDA; Protein Content of Common Food, The On-Off Effect, and PD Quiz, courtesy of the Boston University Medical Center/American Parkinson's Disease Association Information and Referral Center.

ACKNOWLEDGMENTS

I WOULD like to thank Dr. Robert Feldman, Dr. Marie St. Hilaire, Cathi Thomas, R.N., and Linda Perry, R.N., of the Boston University Hospital staff and the Boston PDA Information and Referral Center for their remarkable and generous help. They kindly allowed me to participate in several sessions of the University Hospital's Day Program for Parkinson's Disease, allowing me to see firsthand the effects of the disease and drug therapy in a clinical setting. More important, these sessions gave me the chance to meet several PD patients, some of the most courageous, optimistic, and compassionate people I've ever had the pleasure to meet. I would like to take this opportunity to thank those patients and the many others I met through the Newton-Wellesley Support Group. I wrote this book with you always in mind.

Suzanne LeVert

CONTENTS

Chapter One

Understanding Parkinson's Disease

Aʟᴀɴ ʀᴇᴍᴇᴍʙᴇʀs quite clearly the day he first noticed that his left hand shook. It was a Monday, the day he was to make a sales presentation he'd spent a month preparing. Sitting quietly at his desk, this 54-year-old businessman felt his hand trembling, slightly but persistently. "I put it down to nerves, fatigue, whatever. I'd been feeling depressed and more tired than usual, but otherwise I was in great physical shape. I was only 54. I didn't give it a second thought—until it kept happening."

For Beth, a 68-year-old retired schoolteacher, the onset of her condition was much more gradual, occurring over the course of more than a year. "I tired easily and moved much more slowly. My gardening chores became more difficult and painful to perform. I thought it was just the price I had to pay for getting on in years," she recalls. "But my husband became alarmed when he saw me dragging my right leg, and he complained that I wasn't smiling as much and that I seemed to be staring off into space all the time. When I noticed that I was sort of shuffling when I walked, I became alarmed, too."

Both Alan and Beth would later be diagnosed as having Parkinson's disease, a degenerative brain disease suffered by about one million Americans, most over the age of 50, and just slightly more men than women. They would learn that certain cells in a part of the brain known as the substantia nigra were dying—cells essential to the process of normal human movement. As the cells of the substantia nigra continue to die off, proper movement and balance deteriorate. But neither of them received the diagnosis of Parkinson's on the first visit to a physician.

"My doctor put me through a complete checkup: blood test, chest x-rays, urinalysis, the works," Alan recounts. "He also asked me endless questions about my work routine, what foods I ate, what kind of stress I was under. Because I was feeling so depressed, he referred me to a psychiatrist, whom I saw for about six or seven months. The psychiatrist prescribed antidepressants, but I still wasn't feeling any better. If anything, I felt worse. Then I went to another neurologist, who said, and I quote, 'Well, it doesn't look like Parkinson's disease anyway.' I guess he said this because I didn't have very pronounced symptoms. In fact, my tremor seemed to disappear whenever I went to the doctor! It took about another year and two other neurologists before the diagnosis of PD was confirmed."

Beth's experience was a bit less complicated, but still involved a number of different tests. "Because of my age and because it seemed to be only my right side that felt odd," Beth recalls, "my doctor wanted to rule out the possibility that I'd had a mild stroke without knowing it. He told me up front that a stroke was highly unlikely, mainly because the symptoms seemed to come on gradually and get worse. But he wanted to make sure."

Although Beth's physician suspected PD almost from the start, he knew it was important to rule out the many other conditions—some common and others quite rare—that might account for Beth's symptoms (see Appendix II). Many people suffer from symptoms similar to those caused by Parkinson's disease, but do not actually have the disease itself. When a patient suffers from another disease that produces parkinsonian symptoms, he or she is said to have secondary Parkinson's disease. The causes of these diseases range from the rare, including the inherited, to those caused by certain drugs or toxins. Classic Parkinson's disease, in which the cells of the substantia nigra are being destroyed for an as-yet-unknown reason, is usually referred to as primary or "idiopathic" Parkinson's disease.

No simple blood test or x-ray will confirm PD: The diagnosis is arrived at primarily through physician observation, the elimination of other diseases as the cause of the symptoms, and finally the patient's response to drugs known to reduce the effects of Parkinson's disease (discussed in Chapter Four).

Although you may receive the diagnosis of PD directly from your primary-care physician—many patients do—both Alan and Beth eventually saw brain specialists as well. Neurologists are trained in the art of deciphering the intricate circuitry of the body's least-understood organ, the brain.

A complete neurological exam is an intense, often time-consuming, but almost never painful, experience. It usually begins with the neurologist taking a thorough medical history. He or she will probably ask what other medical conditions you have and what drugs you may be taking, your history of childhood diseases, and if you have had any accidents that involved head or spinal injury. You also will be asked about your family's medical history, especially that of first-tier relatives such as parents, grandparents, siblings, and children, and second-tier relatives such as aunts, uncles, and cousins. This information may help the neurologist rule out some inherited conditions, such as Wilson's disease, that may resemble Parkinson's disease.

Then the doctor performs the physical exam. When a motor (movement) disorder such as Parkinson's disease is suspected, the neurologist will pay special attention to your muscles: how they contract, their strength, and their tone (their resistance to passive movement). The doctor will most likely use the reflex hammer not only in the usual places, such as your knee and elbows, and ankles, but perhaps on your jaw and in other places as well. Every muscle has a reflex, even those that control chewing and swallowing.

Eye movements are studied because the neurologist can tell many things about the function of your nervous system by studying how your eyes move from side to side and up and down. In Parkinson's disease and in some of the diseases that resemble it, there may be a limitation in eye movement—a subtle limitation of which you may not be aware.

Next, the neurologist often likes to see how you move about, how you open and close your hands, tap your feet, how you stand, walk down a hallway, sit back down in your chair. Many neurologists, especially when they suspect PD, will request a sample of your handwriting. In addition, the doctor will take special note of what we think of as body language: Do you cross your legs often or casually brush hair from your face? How often do you blink? Do you smile, frown, or otherwise show emotion when you are speaking or listening? Even the way you get dressed after the exam is data for the doctor's calculations.

Your memory, your ability to do simple mathematical equations, and the sophistication of your abstract reasoning may also be measured at this time. One test for mental function requires you to spell a five-letter word such as "world" forward and backward. This test requires not only rote learning but the ability to juggle things in your mind, remember them, and rearrange them.

Don't be surprised if the exam involves a bit of philosophy as well. To measure your powers of abstract thinking, the neurologist may ask you to interpret a proverb or cliche: What does "A rolling stone gathers no moss" mean to you? for instance. Of course, no right or wrong answer exists to such a question, but how you describe your reaction to it may tell the doctor a great deal about the way your brain is functioning.

More than likely, and again to rule out other conditions that may account for your symptoms, other medical tests may be required. One of the most useful is magnetic resonance imaging, or MRI, which has replaced the computerized axial tomogram, otherwise known as the CAT or, preferably, the CT scan. First introduced in 1984, the MRI scan has become an invaluable medical tool. Hundreds of times more detailed than the ordinary x-ray, MRI scanning can be used to see inside any of the body's organs, including the brain.

The MRI scan is a simple, completely painless procedure, although a few rare patients experience claustrophobia after being placed within the scanner. You'll lie flat on a special table as a powerful magnetic field is created around you. Special radio-frequency waves are pulsed through the field. A detector will pick up changes in the field as the radio waves pass through your brain, then feed the data about tissue density into a computer for analysis. A picture of the result is displayed on a computer screen. The test takes about 20 to 30 minutes and will detect any tumors, cysts, abscesses, or other problems that may be causing your motor dysfunction. Invaluable information on previous, unsuspected strokes may also be obtained.

To rule out brain damage from injury or other neurological disorders not detected on the MRI, the neurologist may request that you have an EEG, an electroencephalogram. If you're scheduled for an EEG, expect to perhaps feel a bit sticky (often glue is used on your scalp) but otherwise completely comfortable. Electrodes are attached to your scalp to record your brain's faint electrical activity. In order to measure how your brain reacts to changes, you may be subjected to flashing lights or noise during the exam.

Other tests may also be administered before your doctor or neurologist determines that you are, indeed, suffering from Parkinson's disease. Although these tests may seem tedious and may be costly, remember that there are other diseases that can be confused with PD. Since PD is a lifelong condition, it is important to rule out these other diseases, which may require special treatment.

One test, called the positron emission tomography, or PET, scan, has provided valuable insights into Parkinson's disease. An extremely sophisticated test, the PET scan can actually detect the presence and location of brain chemicals, something once possible only through the removal of the brain for biochemical analysis. In fact, it may be possible for a PET scan to detect a loss of dopamine—the brain chemical missing or in short supply in the brain of a Parkinson's disease patient—*before* symptoms of Parkinson's disease are apparent. Unfortunately, PET scan equipment is very expensive, costing millions of dollars, and the test is currently available at just a few research centers throughout the world.

Eventually, both Alan and Beth were told by their neurologists that they were indeed suffering from Parkinson's disease. Although their initial symptoms were completely different, each had enough of the cardinal signs of PD that their doctors felt confident that PD was the underlying cause. Alan's shaking hand, depression and exhaustion, and the stiffness in Beth's right side, the dragging of her foot, and her lack of facial expressions were all caused by the same disease.

The Parkinson's Disease Syndrome

As stated earlier, no specific blood test or x-ray will establish Parkinson's disease as a definitive diagnosis. All of Alan's and Beth's tests came back negative: no viruses, tumors, or strokes were causing their symptoms. Apart from ruling out other diseases, what determined the positive diagnosis of PD for Alan and Beth were their own apt descriptions of their symptoms combined with the observations made by their doctors.

Because of this diagnostic process, misdiagnoses can, and often do, occur. Most general practitioners see just two or three new PD patients in an entire year, and even neurologists can be confused by PD's subtle symptoms. Like Alan, you may even find yourself on a psychiatrist's couch for a time before a proper diagnosis is made.

This may be frustrating to both patient and doctor. In the past, it was unimportant as to the length of time it took to diagnose Parkinson's disease because no therapy was available that would affect its progression or severity. Today, although there remains no cure for this progressive brain disease, the advent of a new drug, called selegiline (Eldepryl or deprenyl), may indeed change the course of the disease (see Chapter Four). Now, waiting years, or even months, to begin therapy for Parkinson's disease is no more acceptable than delaying the diagnosis and treatment of a tumor.

One reason this book is being written is to help physicians and patients alike learn as much as possible about PD so that its signs and symptoms are recognized early and treatment started soon. The damage Parkinson's disease does to the brain causes myriad problems related to movement and behavior, some obvious and others more subtle. PD can, in time, result in some patients becoming completely akinetic (totally immobile). In others, few overt manifestations of the disease are present for many years. Most people who suffer from PD come to their physicians with moderate complaints which may progress, slowly or quickly depending on the individual, over a number of years.

It is important to state again—and it will be repeated several times throughout this book—that Parkinson's disease affects each

Primary and Secondary Symptoms of Parkinson's Disease

Cardinal Signs of Parkinson's Disease

- Tremor
- Rigidity (stiffness)
- Bradykinesia (decreased movement)
- Postural instability (unsteadiness, falling)

Secondary Signs of Parkinson's Disease

- Gait disturbances
- Dexterity and coordination difficulties
- Freezing
- Speech and swallowing difficulties
- Visual symptoms
- Depression
- Dementia
- Pain and sensory discomfort
- Sexual difficulty
- Blood pressure changes
- Dermatological changes
- Gastrointestinal and urinary difficulty

patient differently, as do the drugs used to treat it. That said, there are hallmark signs of Parkinson's disease. One or more of these signs are always present in a PD patient.

Cardinal Signs of Parkinson's Disease

Resting Tremor: Tremor, such as the one Alan experienced, occurs in about half to three-quarters of all parkinsonians. It appears most often in the hands and feet, and occasionally may also involve the head, neck, face, lips, tongue, or jaw. The shaking is regular and rhythmic, with a frequency of about 4 to 6 beats per second. In the beginning, the tremor may be worse on one side of the body than the other and the tremor may vary at different times of the day. Physical or emotional stress may also cause tremor to become worse.

"Sometimes I don't even realize my hand is shaking until someone else points it out," says Joe, a patient who has had Parkinson's disease for about 10 years, in describing the uncontrollable tremor that mainly affects his left leg and hand. "A few years ago, I could make it stop if I really concentrated. Now, it's gotten so that I have tremor most of the time, especially in between doses of medication. Sometimes I call myself the 'Shake, rattle, and roll man!' "

Rigidity: Beth's very first symptom was a feeling of stiffness in her right side. "I thought I'd overworked the muscles in my leg, somehow, or slept in the wrong position. But it never went away."

What Beth is experiencing is commonly referred to as rigidity. When your muscles are rigid, they are constantly tensed in a state of sustained contraction—much more tense than the average muscle—even when they should be relaxed. This tension usually is perceived by the patient as stiffness or achiness, and it is the physician who labels it rigidity.

The doctor does this by performing a simple test: After first asking a patient to relax his or her muscles, the doctor then flexes the patient's arm or leg. The resistance to the movement felt by the doctor is known as rigidity. If the arm moves smoothly but with stiffness, the condition is termed *lead-pipe rigidity*, because it resembles the way it would feel to bend a lead pipe. If the arm catches along the path of the flexion, the way a ratchet would in a machine, the doctor might term it *cogwheeling rigidity*. This cogwheeling effect is thought to be caused by a tremor, deep within the muscles and not always visibly apparent, superimposed over the increased tone of the muscle.

Rigidity in Parkinson's disease involves all voluntary muscles, therefore affecting many different activities and body functions. Restricted movement of the arms and legs, evident when the patient is walking with the arms held at the sides and not swinging, is the most obvious result of rigidity, but proper breathing, eating and swallowing, and speech also may be hampered. Beth's poverty of facial expression, first noticed by her husband, is a sign of rigidity. In fact, many patients have a masklike stare, produced by the immobilization of facial muscles and reduction in eye-blinking frequency.

Margaret, a 65-year-old patient diagnosed with PD five years ago, describes rigidity this way: "Rigidity makes me feel as if I haven't had a good stretch in about a hundred years and won't be able to take one for another hundred! I'm tight as a drum, and every movement is difficult."

Bradykinesia: From the Latin *brady* (slow) and *kinesia* (movement), this term describes the often frustratingly long time it takes person with PD to walk, to sit down, or to perform other ordinary movements. In addition to his tremor, Joe suffers from increasing bradykinesia. He describes it this way: "I'm one of the few men I know who loves to relax in a hot bath—I always have. I used to be able to start the bath water, go pour myself a glass of wine, grab a book, get undressed, and get back in time to shut off the tap and jump right in. Now, if I did that, I'd have a flood for sure! Now I get everything ready before I turn on the water. If I'm having a good day, I just have time to get undressed before the tub is full."

For some patients, this slowness affects not only movement but speech and even thought as well. The fact that a PD sufferer may not make certain semiautomatic gestures, such as crossing the legs or scratching the forehead, is also an aspect of bradykinesia.

Postural Instability: Standing up straight, picking up your feet and gently swinging your arms while you walk, being able to right yourself if bumped, are all movements that most of us perform without much conscious thought. You also know instinctively where in space your body is—you don't have to "remember" to uncross your legs before you stand, for instance, your body automatically responds. Some parkinsonians, however, lose these so-called postural reflexes and fall easily.

Generally speaking, some aspect of one or more of these four cardinal signs of PD will be present in a patient. Sometimes a patient will display few parkinsonian symptoms at first, but instead will experience one or more secondary manifestations of the disease. Most often, these secondary signs develop in patients who first experience one of the cardinal signs. Again, not every patient will experience these symptoms, nor may they be experienced exactly as described here.

Secondary Signs of Parkinson's Disease

Gait Disturbances: Many patients with PD develop a stooped, slightly bent posture and tend to propel themselves forward while walking, a syndrome known as festination. Festination consists of an acceleration and abbreviation of movement and, in some patients, of thought as well. Some patients complain of actually feeling "in a hurry" against their will. Some patients may shuffle as they walk, as Beth does, or may have trouble turning around quickly. Together with the loss of postural reflexes, such gait disturbances often lead to dangerous falls, one of the most disabling results of Parkinson's disease. Some doctors believe that gait disturbances result from a combination of rigidity, bradykinesia, and postural instability, while others feel it is a separate symptom.

Dexterity and Coordination Difficulties: A failing tennis serve, increasing golf scores, worsening handwriting, all are among the many signs that Parkinson's disease may be affecting your manual dexterity. These changes may result from a combination of rigidity and bradykinesia or may be a separate phenomenon. When your doctor watches you dress or undress during your examination, it is so that he or she can observe how you manipulate the buttons on your shirt or tie your shoelaces, tasks that require fine motor coordination. Many times, patients first complain of increasingly illegible handwriting: typically, the problem consists of a script that gets smaller and harder to read the longer one writes, called micrographia. That's why your physician may ask you for a handwriting sample during your examination.

Freezing: Patients with Parkinson's disease can experience sudden, involuntary arrest of voluntary movement, a "freezing in one's tracks," so to speak. Although freezing is usually considered a feature of bradykinesia (slowness of movement), it may be a separate phenomenon that can occur independent of other PD symptoms. Characterized by an inability to initiate movement or carry out repetitious acts such as finger tapping or even speaking, freezing is most disabling when it affects walking. Patients feel as if their feet are virtually stuck to the floor, suddenly and often unpredictably. Many patients are particularly prone to freezing when they approach a door or when they turn.

Speech and Swallowing Dysfunction: Patients may complain of slurred, whispered speech, even in the early stages of Parkinson's disease. Others may find that their speech is becoming monotonous or lacking in emotional expression. These symptoms are due to the involvement of the muscles that are used in creating speech, from the diaphragm and throat to the lips and tongue. As some of the muscles that control speech are also involved in swallowing, some patients may complain of swallowing difficulty and may occasionally choke on some foods or pills. Swallowing difficulty is rarely a problem early in the disease.

Visual Symptoms: Patients usually do not complain of visual difficulties because PD does not affect the optic nerves, the nerves that receive visual impressions. Because PD can affect the muscles that move the eyes, however, some patients complain of having difficulty reading. In addition, some drugs that are used to treat PD, particularly the class of drugs called anticholinergic agents, may constrict the pupils, causing blurry vision. A decrease in the number of times per minute patients blink their eyes may lead to other vision-related problems. The normal "windshield wiper effect" of blinking—the wiping away of debris such as dust, smoke, or other irritants—is lost. Conjunctivitis (inflammation of the mucous membrane that covers the front of the eye and lines the inside of the eyelids) may result.

Depression: Serious psychological diseases often occur in Parkinson's disease and chief among them is depression. Although some symptoms of depression are related to the dramatically altered self-image the patient has when faced with the realities of a chronic illness, the occurrence of depression is higher in PD patients than in equally disabled patients with other diseases. This leads physicians to consider that PD also causes changes in the brain's chemistry that result in depression. Depression may occur early or late in PD and may range from mild to severe (requiring hospitalization).

Dementia: The term dementia refers to the progressive loss of memory and other intellectual functions, along with associated changes in behavior and personality. Dementia is the most extreme of the mental changes that occur in PD and is much more common in older (ages 70 and over) than in younger patients—as many as 30 percent of patients in the older age group develop dementia. Alzheimer's disease, which affects about 15 percent of the population over 65, is considered a form of dementia. In some PD patients, the occurrence of dementia may represent the coincidental development of Alzheimer's disease.

In most PD patients, however, the dementia is caused by disease progression. The occurrence of dementia makes treatment of PD more difficult because some of the drugs that improve the motor symptoms of PD (tremor, rigidity, bradykinesia) usually aggravate dementia.

Commonly, patients with PD will display other symptoms such as personality changes, loss of initiative, and fearfulness. However, these changes, although disturbing, do not mean the patient necessarily will develop dementia later in the course of the disease.

The fact that younger patients appear to respond better to medication and exhibit fewer mental changes than their older counterparts has led some scientists to feel that there may be two separate diseases: In younger patients, PD tends to be primarily a motor disease, while in many older patients, PD is both a motor disease and a disease causing disturbances of cognition and emotion.

Pain and Sensory Discomfort: Although pain is rarely a symptom of PD itself, it may be a side effect of medication. Muscle cramps, stiffness, and spasms are the most common complaints. Dystonias, or prolonged spasms, are sometimes painful and usually occur in the muscles of the shoulder, neck, trunk, and calves. Numbness, tingling, and a burning sensation can occur during any stage of the disease, even before motor function is impaired or the disease is diagnosed.

Sexual Difficulty: Every aspect of sexual activity—from initial arousal to orgasm—involves the nervous system, the part of your body that PD most affects. Many PD patients, therefore, experience sexual dysfunction at some point during the course of the disease. While some difficulties may be related to the effects of PD on the nervous system, others result from the mood swings, anxiety, and frustration experienced by some people suffering from a chronic illness. Some difficulties may be caused by the drugs used to treat PD.

Blood Pressure Changes: Occasionally, the part of the brain that controls the activity of the sympathetic nerves, which regulate the heart and blood vessels, may be affected in PD. If the involvement of the sympathetic nervous system (which is part of the autonomic nervous system) is sufficiently severe, low blood pressure may result. Postural hypotension—a drop in blood pressure upon standing—may occur and be experienced as dizziness or lightheadedness. Occasionally, some of the anti-Parkinson drugs may aggravate the postural hypotension and the patient may faint upon standing.

Dermatological Changes: Dermatitis, a type of eczema, is a common side effect of PD. It is characterized by scaly, oily skin, especially around the eyebrows, forehead, eyelids, or nose. It is caused by excess oil being secreted by the sebaceous glands, secondary to the involvement of the autonomic nervous system.

Gastrointestinal and Urinary Dysfunction: Bowel and bladder complaints are common among PD patients. Slowness of movement may affect the muscles that control the bowels, thereby slowing the transit of feces. Constipation, therefore, may be a common and recurrent problem for many patients. This condition is exacerbated if the PD sufferer has difficulty chewing and swallowing and therefore neglects eating enough roughage or drinking enough water. Some anti-Parkinson disease medications—particularly the anticholinergics (see Chapter Four)—may also aggravate constipation. Less frequently, there may be some sluggishness of the bladder musculature so that urination may also be slowed. There may also be difficulty in properly emptying out the bladder, and the patient may thus have to void again immediately after urinating.

Who Gets Parkinson's Disease?

At the beginning of this chapter, you met two people, a man in his mid-50s and a woman in her late 60s, who had PD. Are Alan and Beth "typical" parkinsonians?

In many ways they are. Scientists and physicians estimate that approximately 20 new cases per 100,000 people are diagnosed each year. By far, the majority of PD patients are, like Alan and Beth, over the age of 50 when they are first diagnosed. In fact, many of PD symptoms resemble, and can be mistaken for, the side effects of the normal aging process. Muscular rigidity, gait hesitation, postural imbalance, and some mental disturbances frequently occur in the sixth or seventh decades of a healthy person's life. Indeed, because the symptoms of PD often come on gradually, normal aging may seem at first to be a logical explanation for the difficulties.

As discussed, establishing the exact onset of symptoms in PD may be difficult, because vague complaints such as slow movement, mild aches and pains, easy fatigability, and depression may appear years before a patient feels ill enough to see a doctor and be diagnosed. It is rare for either Parkinson's disease patients or their doctors to be able to pinpoint exactly when PD started. Beth cannot recall, for example, when weeding her garden first caused her hands to ache, or when her leg began to drag. Moreover, by the time she felt these symptoms, the disease process had been ongoing for quite some time.

A majority of parkinsonians experience tremor as their first symptom, and most parkinsonians—more than 75 percent—experience tremor to a greater or lesser extent at some point during the course of their disease. Feelings of general muscle weakness and mood swings are also common among PD patients. Alan's depression and exhaustion are also common first symptoms.

On the other hand, Alan and Beth are not "typical" parkinsonians because Parkinson's disease affects every individual differently. No doctor can reliably predict how fast or far PD will progress, what symptoms will be experienced, or how a patient will respond to treatment. In effect, there is no such thing as a "typical" Parkinson's disease patient at all.

Although the majority of patients are over the age of 50, PD also is diagnosed in patients in their teens, 20s, 30s, and 40s. Unfortunately, reliable statistics on exactly who in the United States has PD are limited, mainly because such data are dependent on an accurate diagnosis. It is not clear if there is more PD among young people or if the apparent increase among young people results from improved diagnoses or heightened awareness about PD among today's population.

It appears that the disease affects men slightly more than women. Why this sexual bias exists is not clear, although it is

---

A Young Parkinson's Patient

Emily Hamilton is one of the youngest Parkinson's disease patients diagnosed. Emily's disease began when she was about 3½ years of age. At that time she exhibited a rather common, but nonspecific, problem among children called "toeing in." Emily's toes would flex and she walked with her toes in this position. At age 5, her printing, which had been good, deteriorated into a scrawl and her walking became more difficult.

Like many adult PD patients, Emily's symptoms fluctuated. In the morning, she could walk and write normally. By late morning, however, she had trouble with these simple activities, and by nightfall she could only crawl. Her left arm was bent at the elbow, her left leg at the knee, and both of her hands would tremble.

Just as many adult diseases have symptoms that resemble Parkinson's disease, so too are there conditions found in children that look like, but are not, Parkinson's disease (see Appendix II). But none of these disorders—except for a rare form of dystonia or altered muscular tone that is seen predominantly in Japan—explained Emily's condition. Instead, it appears that she, like her adult fellow sufferers, has Parkinson's disease. She too went through more than one series of tests before she was diagnosed with Parkinson's disease in January of 1989. Once treated with medication, however, most of her symptoms disappeared. A bright and optimistic young lady, Emily faces a future of uncertainty with remarkable courage.

possible that either male hormones aggravate or female hormones protect against the process that causes PD.

Some statistics indicate that African-Americans have a lower incidence of PD than Caucasians. It may be that African-Americans are somehow physically protected from the disease or, alternatively, that their limited access to quality health care and neurology specialists has distorted the true picture of Parkinson's disease in the United States.

Hugh, a 24-year-old marketing executive from a large southern city, received his diagnosis two years ago—the same week he earned his college diploma. "My first reaction was one of relief, to tell you the truth. I was convinced I had a brain tumor!" he recalls with a laugh. "It all started when I was in my junior or senior year in high school. My lower legs started feeling weak and trembly. And they kept getting worse. Then my handwriting started getting smaller. People kept asking me to repeat things and to speak more slowly." Hugh paused to recall his two-year odyssey. "I went to about six doctors before I got my diagnosis. I even had a spinal tap, which was one of the most painful and humiliating experiences I've ever had. All the while neurologists kept telling me, 'You can't have Parkinson's disease, you're too young.' But it turns out I do, and as daunting and humbling as it is, it's good to know. Now I can deal with it for what it is."

Once they were diagnosed, Hugh, Alan, and Beth were told the proverbial "bad news and good news." The bad news is that, as yet, no cure for Parkinson's disease has been found. The good news is that there are effective drugs that will help them remain healthy, active people for many years and that there are drugs that may slow down the progression of the disease (see Chapter Four).

"When I first heard the diagnosis, my heart sank. My best friend's father had Parkinson's disease back in the 1950s and he became almost completely paralyzed. I was so afraid that that would happen to me," Beth declared. "But then my doctor told me about a Parkinson's patient he'd been treating for more than 15 years. At the age of 65, she still drove her car, tended her garden, and played bridge with her friends every Wednesday afternoon."

Indeed, the drugs used to treat the symptoms of Parkinson's disease can increase mobility, help stop tremors, and restore some flexibility and agility. Currently, anti-Parkinson drugs allow most patients to maintain relatively healthy and normal lives for about 5 to 20 years after diagnosis, depending on how fast the disease progresses in the particular individual. For patients in their 20s, 30s, and 40s, or for even younger patients like Emily, the future is less certain. However, the introduction of drugs like selegiline (also known as Eldepryl or deprenyl) may slow the progression of the disease by as much as 50 percent—a ray of hope for younger Parkinson patients.

Discovering what causes this disease and learning exactly how the brain is affected by it will go a long way both in developing therapies for patients of all ages and stages of the disease and in finding a cure. In the next two chapters, we'll see how far scientific research has come during the past two centuries in giving us a road map of the brain and the way it misfunctions in Parkinson's disease.

Chapter Two

The Story of Parkinson's Disease

To BOTH observers and sufferers of Parkinson's disease, uncooperative, unresponsive muscles appear to be causing the disease's most troublesome symptoms: the hand that won't stop shaking, the leg that simply won't take another step, the face that no longer breaks into a ready smile. But in fact, Parkinson's disease is not a muscle disorder at all. Indeed, the muscles of a PD patient, when properly exercised (as will be discussed in Chapter Five), will remain healthy throughout the course of the disease.

Most of the vast and complicated nervous system remains intact in a PD patient, including the nerves that transmit messages to and from the spinal cord to the body's muscles and organs. Parkinson's disease arises from a disorder in a small part of the brain called the substantia nigra, or "black substance." In the substantia, the large pigmented neurons (nerve cells) undergo a mysterious degeneration, depriving the brain of a chemical called dopamine that is manufactured in the substantia nigra and that is crucial to proper human movement.

The cells of the substantia nigra connect with cells in another area of the brain called the striatum, which help to initiate and control movement and balance. Messages pass between the cells of the substantia nigra and the cells in the striatum through the aid of dopamine, which acts as a neurotransmitter, helping to transmit messages from one nerve cell to another.

As the dopamine-producing neurons in the substantia nigra die, the amount of dopamine in the striatum decreases. Without dopamine, the work of the striatum is interrupted, causing many of the symptoms of Parkinson's disease.

The mechanisms and chemistry involved in movement and behavior, and how they malfunction in PD, are extremely complex. The simple summary given above, although far from complete, reflects centuries of research. As the science of medicine has evolved, so too has knowledge of the brain and its circuitry.

The History of Parkinson's Disease

Since before the time of Christ, physicians and other observers of the human condition have described people with tremors, with stooped posture, and with the rapid, off-balance walk called festination. Whether all the people observed with these symptoms actually had Parkinson's disease, of course, will never be known. Slowly but surely, however, medical science began to define and delineate the symptoms of PD and, eventually, its underlying cause within the brain.

Although descriptions of what may be PD symptoms can be found in texts written more than two thousand years ago, the first important record was made in the second century A.D. by the great Greek physician Galen. Galen's accomplishments were many: It was he who made the discovery that blood and not air was carried by our arteries, for instance. Galen also developed many modern research methods, such as animal dissection and experimentation, which set the standard for medical science for centuries.

Galen was also a keen observer of symptoms: He was the first to make distinctions between different kinds of tremor and may have described the tremor of PD. However, there is much debate as to whether what he described was indeed PD. Another early researcher who may have described PD was Leonardo da Vinci.

During the fourteenth century, an Italian physician named Franciscus de la Boe made another discovery about tremor: He claimed that the tremor experienced when the body was moving or performing some activity like writing or walking was markedly different from that experienced when the body was still. Indeed, we now recognize that an action tremor usually has a different cause and requires different treatment than a resting tremor. Although action tremors may occur in PD, the resting tremor is so much more common that it is considered a hallmark sign of PD.

William Shakespeare also contributed to our knowledge of tremor. In *Measure for Measure* (Act I, Scene iii), he differentiated between the shaking associated with fevers or disease and that associated with old age.

By far, the most important early contribution to the story of PD was made by a 62-year-old London surgeon in 1817. When James Parkinson's "Essay on the Shaking Palsy" was published, the distinct syndrome of symptoms that now bears his name was described in depth for the first time. In this manuscript, he recounts his observations and examinations of just six patients, one of whom he merely watched walk down a crowded London street. Parkinson concentrated on PD's most obvious symptom, tremor. He saw that in his patients the tremor would start as an intermittent trembling of one limb; then this tremor eventually became uncontrollable. He also noticed in the patients that "by suddenly changing the posture [the tremor] is for a time stopped in that limb to commence, generally in less than a minute, in one of the legs or in the arm of the other side."

Like Galen centuries before, Parkinson made a distinction between the condition then known as the shaking palsy (*paralysis agitans*) and the involuntary movements associated with other diseases, such as epilepsy. In addition, Parkinson drew attention to the distinction between the trembling of paralysis agitans and the trembling due to the excess intake of alcohol, tea, and coffee. Parkinson stressed the association of paralysis (palsy) with tremor, but indicated that, at least in the patients he examined, paralysis came on quite slowly and was never complete, even in the advanced stages of disease. While Parkinson used the word paralysis to describe his patients' poverty of movement, we now call this symptom bradykinesia. Parkinson also made the essential link between festination, stooped posture, stiffness, and tremor; for the first time, these seemingly disparate symptoms were considered to be part of the same condition.

After the publication of Parkinson's essay, other scientists and physicians built upon the observations made in his text. Jean-Martin Charcot, a French physician, worked in Paris in the middle to late 1800s. It was Charcot who insisted that the disease be named after Parkinson. According to Charcot, rigidity, stooped posture, and slow movement were just as important as, and could be present separately from, tremor.

After Parkinson's disease was defined, physicians searched for its cause. Just where in the body's complex and as yet largely unmapped brain and nervous system was the problem? Although the physical changes in the body are marked, the anatomical changes in the brain are slight, and it was 100 years after Parkinson's description that the damage to the substantia nigra was discovered. Prior to this, the disease was attributed to a number of causes, including stroke, diseases of the spinal cord, or even to muscle or nerve abnormalities. Some even considered it to be psychosomatic or psychopathic in origin.

Encephalitis Lethargica

During the 1920s, an Austrian neurologist named Constantin von Economo studied a viral epidemic that had plagued communities, particularly in central Europe and the United States, since about 1915. The virus caused encephalitis, or inflammation of the brain. Because one of its primary symptoms was prolonged sleepiness, this epidemic encephalitis was also known as *encephalitis lethargica*. Nearly 50 percent of all victims of this virus, about 500,000 people worldwide, died during the initial phase of the illness.

In addition to sleepiness, the surviving patients developed problems with eye movements, had difficulty swallowing, and experienced changes in personality and behavior. Many also became emotionally withdrawn and passive. After about six months, most of the acute symptoms eased, but many patients remained disabled, with tremors, muscle rigidity, marked mental changes, and other problems. Others apparently made full recoveries, only to be plagued with symptoms a few years later. This is the disorder decribed by Oliver Sacks in his book, *Awakenings*.

The similarities in the symptoms and disabilities between postencephalitic patients and idiopathic (cause unknown) Parkinson's disease patients were remarkable; in fact, a new syndrome called *postencephalitic parkinsonism* was designated and was the most common type of parkinsonism—especially in young adults—seen by physicians during the 1930s and 1940s.

Marked differences between the two conditions existed as well, however. Most postencephalitic patients experienced what are called oculogyric crises, in which the head and eyes turned up—as if to look at the ceiling—for hours at a time. Rapid facial and body movements and obsessive-compulsive rituals were other postencephalitic symptoms not common to patients with idiopathic Parkinson's disease. In addition, the rate of progression of symptoms was usually much less in postencephalitic parkinsonism than in Parkinson's disease.

Scientists attempted to identify the virus that caused encephalitis, but with no success. Although other viruses can cause encephalitis, so far no other type of encephalitis has been found to produce similar parkinsonian symptoms in its victims. Nevertheless, the epidemic did raise the possibility that idiopathic Parkinson's disease, like its cousin, could also be caused by an infectious agent. Could a virus or a toxin cause Parkinson's disease? That is a question as yet unanswered.

Brain Anatomy and Parkinson's Disease

Meanwhile, the science of neurology was advancing apace. By the end of the 1800s, many brain structures had been identified and their functions, if not confirmed, at least suspected. In 1915, nearly a century after James Parkinson's landmark essay, a medical student named von Tretiakoff claimed that the substantia nigra, a tiny patch of darkly colored cells, was the culprit in this movement disorder. Autopsies performed on the brains of patients with Parkinson's disease showed one striking abnormality: a marked decrease in the number of substantia nigra cells. Precisely why this decrease caused patients to tremble, have stooped posture, or become stiff would not be known for another fifty years.

An extraordinarily complicated and intricate structure, the work of the brain comprises millions of complex electrical and chemical actions and reactions taking place every second. Everything we are, what we think, what foods we like, how fast we run, who we love—all of these qualities and activities are stimulated by the brain and its network of nerve cells distributed throughout the body.

FIGURE 1.
THE BRAIN AND PARKINSON'S DISEASE.

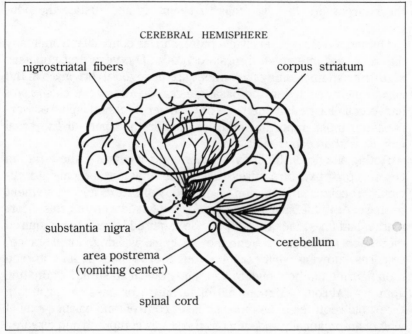

CEREBRAL HEMISPHERE

nigrostriatal fibers

corpus striatum

substantia nigra

cerebellum

area postrema
(vomiting center)

spinal cord

The basic unit of your entire nervous system is the neuron, a tiny cell less than 1/100 of an inch in diameter. Your brain and nervous system consist of millions of neurons dispersed throughout the body. Through their work, your brain receives and responds to messages from your body's internal organs as well as from the outside environment. The normal functioning of the body depends upon the proper reception and response to stimuli.

Different groups of neurons perform different functions: Sensory neurons transmit messages about sights, sounds, and other stimuli from the environment to the brain. Motor neurons transmit messages to and from the spinal cord and muscles, glands, and other body parts. Within the brain itself, some neurons are organized into subsets of specialized cells, each of which is believed to control certain activities. The brainstem, for instance, is a group of neurons that regulate autonomic (automatic) bodily functions such as breathing, blood pressure, and heart rate. Interneurons, the most numerous type of brain cell, shuttle signals back and forth between various parts of the brain and spinal cord. Surrounding the neurons are the glial cells that support and sustain the neurons.

Human movement, in all its complexity, is controlled from many different, but interrelated, brain centers. The very first impulses initiating and fine-tuning movement are believed to originate in the cerebral cortex and in the basal ganglia, several large clusters of nerve cells located at the base of each cerebral hemisphere. Perhaps the most important and best understood part of the basal ganglia is the corpus striatum.

Acting as one of the body's motor control centers, the striatum (made up of two structures called the putamen and caudate nucleus) receives information about body position and movement from several different parts of the brain. It integrates this information and fine-tunes the commands required to initiate a required movement. Picking up your foot to begin walking, for instance, requires knowing what position your foot is in to begin with and then figuring out how high to lift it and how far to step. Negotiating your way through a room full of furniture or passing through a threshold requires even more finesse, control, and balance—all of which, automatically and subconsciously, is computed and directed from within the striatum. The striatum is also responsible for maintaining normal muscle tone and, therefore, proper body posture.

After the striatum makes its computations, it sends impulses to other parts of the brain's motor control system. From there, messages are transmitted to the spinal cord, then through the peripheral nerves to the muscles themselves, through several complicated nerve circuits.

Integral to this process is the substantia nigra, which lies beneath the striatum in a part of the brain called the midbrain. About the size of a fingertip, the substantia nigra has long been the focus of Parkinson's disease research. Even before von Tretiakoff published his findings in 1915, autopsies had indicated the involvement of this tiny patch of cells in Parkinson's disease. Later, the brains of encephalitis lethargica victims, examined during the 1920s, showed the same abnormalities. Then, in 1939, a German physician named Hassler published a study confirming von Tretiakoff's findings.

Nevertheless, scientists did not understand the significance of the changes observed in the substantia nigra until the 1950s, after major advances in brain chemistry had occurred.

The Synapse

Until the end of the nineteenth century, scientists thought the brain consisted not of individual cells, like other parts of the body, but was instead a continuous mass of tissue. It wasn't until an Italian anatomist, Camillo Golgi, developed a stain that exposed an entire neuron, allowing its anatomy and its processes to be examined, that the scientific community accepted that the brain was made up of billions of separate, distinct neurons.

Golgi's stain revealed that a typical neuron consists of a cell body and a number of fibers extending from it. The neuron transmits information to other nerve cells by sending information out of its cell body through just one of its hairlike fibers, the axon. All the other fibers extending from the cell body *receive* information from other cells. These receptors are called dendrites.

The neuron is the functional unit of the brain. It receives information, in the form of electrical impulses, at its dendrites. The impulse passes through its cell body, then out its axon to other neurons. The axon typically divides into a number of small fibers that end in terminals, each of which forms what is called a synapse with another cell. The synapse is actually a space between the axon terminal of one neuron and the dendrite receptor of another.

Just as a car requires oil to allow its gears to shift properly, nerve cells need certain chemicals in order for this intricate circuitry to function properly. These chemicals, called neurotransmitters, provide the connection between the axon of one neuron and the dendrite of another. In essence, neurotransmitters allow electrical impulses to pass from one cell across the synapse to another.

When a neuron is first stimulated, it sets off an electrical current, which releases neurotransmitters stored near the neuron's axon terminals. These chemicals flow across the synapses to stimulate the next neuron in the nerve fiber; the process continues until the message is received by the proper center. Without the presence of neurotransmitters, neurons cannot send appropriate messages to other parts of the brain.

In fact, the synaptic transmission is the event behind all the doings of the nervous system. Every human activity, from orchestrating a sneeze to composing a symphony, is accomplished through a series of synaptic transmissions. The human brain, composed of perhaps 100 billion neurons, has at least 10 *trillion* synapses. An individual neuron may have several thousand alone, each of them requiring a proper neurotransmitter.

The Biochemistry of Neurotransmission

During the 1950s, a new technique—in fact, a high-tech cousin to the one discovered by Golgi in the last century—allowed neurotransmitters to be measured and observed for the first time. A group of Swedish researchers, led by Arvid Carlsson, applied this staining technique to the substantia nigra, the striatum, and other parts of the basal ganglia. What they found was large amounts of the neurotransmitter called dopamine. Dopamine, they discovered, was produced in the darkly pigmented cells of the substantia nigra, then transmitted to the striatum, where it allowed the complex computations concerning body movement to take place. Two other Swedish researchers, A. Dahlstron and K. Fuxe, were the first to delineate the nigrostriatal fibers: the pathway from the substantia nigra to the striatum.

Suddenly, the pathology of Parkinson's disease became clear. In a healthy brain, the substantia nigra produces enough dopamine to allow the striatum to perform its complicated activities. But in the brain of a parkinsonian, dopamine-producing cells are destroyed and the striatum does not receive enough dopamine to fuel the millions of synaptic transmissions required to create smooth, continuous voluntary movement or maintain proper posture or muscle tone. The deficiency of dopamine in the striatum of PD patients was discovered by a Hungarian and an Austrian researcher, O. Hornykiewicz and W. Birkenmayer.

Dopamine is not the only neurotransmitter found in the basal

FIGURE 2.
THE SYNAPSE.

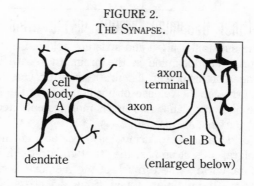

Two communicating neurons are shown here. Cell A is shown complete with its three parts labeled: dendrites, cell body, and axon with its terminal. Cell B is shown in part, with its dendrites located close by the terminal of Cell A.

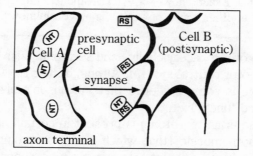

The synapse between Cell A and Cell B. Neurotransmitter molecules (NT) are located inside Cell A. One neurotransmitter molecule has been released from Cell A and is attached to a receptor site (RS) on Cell B. This interaction of NT and RS is the chemical means whereby Cell A can transfer information to Cell B.

Other Dopamine Circuits in the Brain

Although the substantia nigra and striatum hold more than three-quarters of all the dopamine in the brain, there are two other systems in need of this powerful neurotransmitter. One circuit uses dopamine to trigger the release of hormones from the hypothalamus and the pituitary gland. Another is more complicated and may be linked to Parkinson's disease.

A group of dopamine-producing cells, located right next to the substantia nigra, project up past the striatum into the frontal lobes of the cerebral cortex where much of the memory, sensory, and thinking areas of the brain are found. Some scientists believe that schizophrenia and other mental illnesses may be connected to an excess of dopamine in this circuit. As you'll learn in Chapter Four, antiparkinsonian drugs devised to replace the dopamine lost in Parkinson's disease often cause hallucinations and other mental disturbances. It is possible that these drugs also cause an overdose of dopamine in the cerebral cortex, resulting in symptoms similar to schizophrenia. Exactly how—or even if—the two dopamine circuits are related in other ways, however, is as yet unknown.

ganglia. Two others, acetylcholine and serotonin, also play roles in the brain's motor control system. Although their roles are not yet defined, there is some evidence that Parkinson's disease affects their level and function, too.

Outside the brain, serotonin is present in certain body tissues, such as smooth muscle (that which controls involuntary movements) and in blood platelets. In the brain, it appears to be involved in the process of sleep. Although its role in body movement is uncertain, serotonin, like dopamine, is found in high concentrations in the cells of healthy basal ganglia.

Acetylcholine is one of the most abundant transmitters in the body. Outside the brain, it is found at the junctions between nerves and muscles and at certain other sites in the autonomic system, such as the heart. Relatively little is known about how acetylcholine works in the brain except that it, too, is found in the basal ganglia. Scientists think that acetylcholine is important for normal intellectual functions, such as learning and memory. A lack of acetylcholine, many believe, contributes in ways yet unknown to Alzheimer's disease.

In addition, acetylcholine is known to be an excitatory substance: An excess of acetylcholine in the brain results in an increased rate of synaptic transmission within the basal ganglia.
Such hyperstimulation of neurons can cause symptoms quite similar to those caused by a depletion of dopamine, particularly tremor
and rigidity.

The involvement of serotonin, acetylcholine, and other neurotransmitters in the activities of the basal ganglia has led many
researchers to the conclusion that, although dopamine insufficiency
is the most obvious problem in Parkinson's disease, the *imbalance*
between several neurotransmitters in the basal ganglia is also of
importance. As we'll see in Chapter Four, drug therapies have
been developed to address these imbalances, as well as to address
the dopamine insufficiency.

One other link in the brain's chain of reactions must be explained
here. Where do neurotranmsitters come from in the first place?
And how are they regulated by the body and the brain? Without
this knowledge, an effective way to restore the brain's biochemical
balance is impossible.

All neurotransmitters, including dopamine and acetylcholine,
must first be synthesized from raw materials in the body. Dopamine, for instance, is made from tyrosine, an amino acid derived
from eating protein-containing foods, such as meat and nuts. An
enzyme, called tyrosine hydroxylase, converts tyrosine into a
chemical called levodopa. Levodopa is then converted into dopamine by another enzyme, dopa decarboxylase.

Like acetylcholine and serotonin, dopamine is also used in other
parts of the body. Some of the tyrosine we absorb is taken up by
the adrenal glands, two hormone-producing structures located on
the surface of the kidneys. In the adrenal glands, the creation of
dopamine from tyrosine takes place just as it does in the brain, but
is then taken one step further. Another enzyme synthesizes the
dopamine into a chemical called norepinephrine.

One of the most powerful and important of the body's transmitters, norepinephrine works on the sympathetic nervous system,
helping to regulate blood pressure, heart rate, breathing, and digestion. As we'll see in Chapter Four, developing a drug that
would increase the amount of dopamine in the brain without increasing the amount of norepinephrine in the body proved to be

quite a challenge. In addition, norepinephrine is synthesized from dopamine in other parts of the brain, including a structure located near the substantia nigra. Called the locus ceruleus (the blue spot), these brain cells are thought to be connected to memory, sleep patterns, and other cognitive activities and require the neurotransmitter norepinephrine to send their messages. Although no definite proof has been found, some researchers believe that a norepinephrine deficit in this structure is somehow related to the memory and sleep problems affecting some PD patients.

A healthy brain has ways to control the amount of neurotransmitters available to the neurons. No matter how much protein you eat, for instance, only a certain amount of tyrosine will be converted into levodopa and then into dopamine. Scientists have been able to produce levodopa outside of the body and it is now the principal anti-Parkinson drug. Levodopa itself, however, does not act as a neurotransmitter. It needs to be converted to dopamine by another chemical process first. It is this synthesis that regulates the amount of dopamine produced in the brain.

Acetylcholine, too, is converted from an amino acid commonly found in foodstuffs. The amino acid, called choline, is found in egg yolks and many different vegetables. After choline-containing foods are digested, the choline passes into the blood and is taken up by neurons. There it combines with other metabolic products to become the neurotransmitter acetylcholine. Excess acetylcholine is inactivated (broken down) by an enzyme called acetylcholinesterase. Without this enzyme, too much acetylcholine would accumulate, leading to an overstimulation of basal ganglia neurons. Drugs have been developed to help this breakdown process take place, thereby inhibiting the activity of the acetylcholine.

After a synapse between two cells has taken place, another enzyme breaks down and disposes of the leftover dopamine. This enzyme is called monoamine oxidase B, or MAO B, and it is present at both the axon terminal of one cell and the dendrite receptor at the other. MAO B is also present in the supporting glial cells. While MAO B is important in preventing the accumulation of dopamine within the neuron, the amount of the enzyme increases with age. It is felt by some researchers that this increase in MAO B may somehow be responsible for the formation of compounds called "free radicals" that may damage neurons. Free radicals are particles that can react with—and damage—the lipid (fat) layers that surround and insulate cells.

If not deactivated, free radicals are capable of damaging otherwise healthy cells. In a healthy brain, the substantia nigra produces an enzyme that neutralizes free radicals that form during the breakdown of dopamine and acetylcholine. However, in the brains of PD patients, that enzyme is severely depleted. Recent research suggests that as PD progresses, some cells of the substantia nigra may be being destroyed by free radicals.

By the end of the 1960s, the general pathology of Parkinson's disease had pretty much been confirmed. The medical community agreed that the problem was caused by a decrease of certain cells of the substantia nigra, which led to a depletion of the neurotransmitter dopamine. Further, the decrease in dopamine caused an imbalance among other neurotransmitters, especially acetylcholine and serotonin.

What science did not know, and still does not know, is the underlying cause of Parkinson's disease. What causes substantia nigra cells to stop producing dopamine in the first place? In the next chapter, you'll read about some of the theories developed to try to explain the cause of this mysterious condition.

Chapter Three

PD: Its Causes and Progression

Thanks to the remarkable advances made in biochemistry, pharmacology, and molecular biology in recent decades, very powerful and effective drugs have been developed to treat Parkinson's disease. These drugs, discussed in depth in Chapter Four, allow patients to lead fairly healthy and active lives for many years after diagnosis.

Despite this wealth of knowledge, no reliable cure for Parkinson's disease exists today. Why? Because although scientists know *what* goes wrong in the brain of a Parkinson's disease patient, they do not know *why* it goes wrong. Exactly what causes the cells of the substantia nigra to stop producing the essential neurotransmitter dopamine continues to mystify neurologists. And discovering the cause is the best hope for developing a cure.

Searching for clues, researchers have looked to patients who suffer from what is called "secondary parkinsonism." These people suffer from parkinsonian symptoms, such as tremor, bradykinesia, and gait problems, but the cause of their condition is, to a larger degree, known. In some cases, the cells of the substantia nigra or the striatum are directly affected, in about the same way they are in idiopathic Parkinson's diseases. In others, the symptoms are caused by damage to another part of the brain.

Secondary Parkinsonism

Vascular Parkinsonism

In order to survive and to function, all neurons depend on oxygen and nutrients brought to them in the bloodstream. Without oxygen, neurons die, and once they die, they often are not replaced. Stop the supply of oxygen for just a few seconds or minutes and permanent brain damage results.

Brain damage caused by lack of blood (and the oxygen it brings) is called a stroke. Any number of disorders can cause a stroke. Two in combination are particularly problematic: high blood pressure and atherosclerosis, also known as hardening of the arteries. In atherosclerosis, a thick, rough deposit of plaque—usually consisting of the fat called cholesterol—forms on the walls of the blood vessels, especially those weakened by the strain of high blood pressure. Eventually, the plaque may totally close off an artery (thrombosis), break off and travel until it wedges itself into a blood vessel in the brain (embolus), or weaken the blood vessels to the breaking point (cerebral hemorrhage). The result of any of these events is the death of brain cells from lack of oxygen.

The location of the stroke and its severity determine its effect upon the patient. The ability to create or understand language is affected by some strokes; in others partial or total paralysis is the result. In some cases, symptoms appear that are easily confused with those of Parkinson's disease.

Like Parkinson's disease, stroke is a disease of the elderly; most strokes occur in people over the age of 60. In fact, the process of aging itself may cause damage to brain vessels: After years of pumping blood to and from the heart and brain, the walls of the vessels may be damaged, attracting fatty deposits that further weaken them. In the brain, thousands of tiny capillaries (the smallest blood vessel) may be so weakened that they begin either to leak blood into surrounding brain tissue (hemorrhage) or to close up. Closure of these small vessels results in small "ministrokes" called lacunes, literally holes in the brain. Most of the lacunes occur in the basal ganglia.

The damage caused by these ministrokes may be subtle, and the patient may be unaware that they are occurring. Often, however, he or she is left with some stiffness and slowness, a tendency to walk with short, shuffling steps, and with some difficulty speaking clearly. In short, they suffer from the very symptoms associated with Parkinson's disease, not surprising since many of the ministrokes also occur in the basal ganglia.

Today, physicians generally have little trouble differentiating between stroke and Parkinson's disease. Usually, the onset of symptoms of stroke, even of small strokes, is rapid, while the symptons of Parkinson's disease evolve over months or years. That was the reason that Beth's doctor ruled out stroke in her case, described in Chapter One. In addition, magnetic resonance imaging also will usually show the damage from ministrokes. And even if the onset is uncertain, the patient suffering from parkinsonism secondary to many small strokes usually does not respond to drugs used to treat idiopathic Parkinson's disease. Unfortunately, however, some patients may have a combination of neurological problems, including both Parkinson's disease and ministrokes. This can further complicate diagnosis and treatment.

Infectious Parkinsonism

As discussed in Chapter Two, a viral epidemic during the 1910s and 1920s caused parkinsonian symptoms in many of its victims. Autopsies found that the virus selectively destroyed the same cells of the substantia nigra as did idiopathic Parkinson's disease.

Viruses are the body's most clever and dangerous enemies. Smaller than bacteria, they can be seen—when they can be seen at all—only under an electron microscope. Viruses can reproduce only in a living cell. After entering the body through breaks in the skin, by being inhaled, or through the blood, they attach themselves to a cell, invade it, and take over the genetic machinery of the cell. Viruses then compel the cell to reproduce more viral particles. The virus keeps reproducing over and over again, until the host cell is overfull and bursts. The host cell dies, and countless viral particles are released to invade other cells. Some diseases caused by viruses are the common cold, measles, polio, and AIDS.

When the encephalitis lethargica virus struck, some neurologists concluded that all cases of PD, past and present, were caused by a similar virus. Autopsy after autopsy, however, failed to uncover such a link, and to this day, no scientific evidence has been found to support the viral theory. Nevertheless, the idea that a virus or other organism from outside the body might be causing the death of cells in the substantia nigra continues to intrigue the medical community. It is an avenue of research still being explored.

Drug-Induced Parkinsonism

The 1950s ushered in a new era in the treatment of psychiatric disorders such as anxiety, depression, and schizophrenia. Once unable to do anything more than control patients' behavior with the use of restraints, physicians could now prescribe drugs that would alleviate many heretofore intractable symptoms.

One of the first tranquilizers prescribed was called resperine, which could also control high blood pressure. One of resperine's unexpected side effects provided another clue to the mystery of Parkinson's disease. Just when other researchers were discovering that substantia nigra cells produced dopamine and that these cells were deficient in Parkinson's disease patients, physicians were finding that some patients taking resperine were developing parkinsonian symptoms, including rigidity and tremor.

What was the relationship between resperine (and other tranquilizers) and Parkinson's disease? Animal research, by Arvid Carlsson and others, showed that resperine and similar drugs caused depletion of neurotransmitters in the brain, including dopamine and serotonin. Other tranquilizers acted in another way: They blocked the receptors for dopamine in the striatum. In either case, striatal synapses integral to human movement and behavior were not able to take place, mimicking the problem in idiopathic PD.

Unlike strokes or virus-induced parkinsonism, both of which destroy brain tissue, drug-induced parkinsonism is reversible. The symptoms appear after several weeks of drug therapy, and usually disappear a few weeks or months after the therapy is stopped.

Drugs like resperine, and other tranquilizers such as haloperidol (Haldol) and chlorpromazine (Thorazine), and the antinauseant

Metoclopromide (reglan), did not cause Parkinson's disease in most patients. But not only did drug-induced parkinsonism confirm the theory that too little dopamine (caused by reserpine) resulted in parkinsonian symptoms, it provided a new avenue of therapy as well. If certain drugs could deplete neurotransmitters, researchers deduced, then other drugs could replace them. If certain drugs kept the receptors in the striatum from receiving dopamine, then others could stimulate them.

One of the most important drug-related clues to the cause of Parkinson's disease was discovered in the late 1970s and early 1980s after several heroin addicts injected themselves with a homemade narcoticlike drug and developed symptoms indistinguishable from idiopathic Parkinson's disease. These addicts rapidly became bradykinetic, rigid, tremulous, and exhibited postural instability, and some became totally immobilized. Unlike drug-induced parkinsonian patients, the symptoms experienced by these addicts were permanent.

The substance with which the addicts had injected themselves was a chemical mistakenly produced in an attempt to create a synthetic form of the narcotic meperidine, or Demerol. The substance, called MPTP (short for N-methyl-4-phenyl-1,2,3,6-tetrahydropyridine) did not itself kill the substantia nigra cells. Once in the body, however, MPTP was converted by enzyme action into another substance called MPP+, which did destroy nigral cells. The enzyme responsible for the conversion was none other than monoamine oxidase B, the same enzyme that breaks down dopamine after it is released during neurotransmission.

W. Langston, T. Tetrud, and P. Ballard connected the injection of MPTP with the development of parkinsonism in the addicts. Then S. Burns and S. Markey were able to demonstrate that MPTP injected into monkeys also caused parkinsonism and that the parkinsonism resulted from the selective destruction of the cells of the substantia nigra. While MPTP-induced parkinsonism is not identical with idiopathic PD, it has provided a valuable animal model of PD and new insights into its causes and progression. Thus it was found that selegiline (Eldepryl), a drug that blocks MAO B, could, if administered before an injection of MPTP, prevent parkinsonism. By blocking MAO B, it slows down the breakdown of dopamine. Selegiline had been used since 1977 as an anti-Parkinson drug, used to extend the efficacy of levodopa, the major anti-Parkinson drug.

Many researchers now believe that it is possible that selegiline, given as soon as possible after the diagnosis of PD is made, may slow the progression of the disease. A large multicentered study called DATATOP, involving more than 800 patients, strongly suggests that selegiline does indeed slow the progression of PD. Ideally, if PD could be diagnosed before symptoms began, the results would be even better. Much research now centers on developing just such means of early diagnosis.

MPTP obviously does not explain the vast majority of PD cases. But understanding the way MPTP worked within the body caused researchers to ask another question: Could similar substances from the outside environment be converted to a toxin that selectively destroys nigral cells?

Idiopathic Parkinson's Disease

As discussed in Chapter One, most patients suffering from PD cannot directly trace their disease to stroke, drugs, or toxins. If not a virus or a toxin, what could be causing their brains to degenerate? A number of theories, none of them universally accepted, have been proposed.

Aging

A certain number of human cells die every day, some of them, including brain cells, never to be replaced. A perfectly normal occurrence, this cell death is the cause of many of the problems related to the aging process: everything from muscle stiffness to small memory lapses can often be attributed to the toll extracted from the human body by the passage of time.

In fact, some researchers believe that if everyone lived to be over 120, we all would eventually develop Parkinson's disease as more and more of our dopamine-producing cells were lost through the normal aging process. If there has been an increase in the number of Parkinson's patients since 1815, when the disease was first defined, it could be related to the fact that the average life expectancy has risen considerably, from about 45 years to about 70 years.

On the other hand, of course, many PD patients are in their 50s, 40s, and even younger—long before aging could be invoked as an explanation for their condition. The possibility that some kind of accelerated aging process is taking place in the brain of PD patients has been considered, but what the process is or how it is activated remains unclear.

Genetics

Many parkinsonians have remarked that they have relatives who either have undiagnosed tremor or have been diagnosed with Parkinson's disease. Most other patients, however, claim no familial link.

The study of the human gene is one of the fastest-growing areas of scientific research. Every day, it seems, a new gene defect or mutation is discovered as a cause for a disease. Recently, for instance, researchers claim to have found a gene mutation that causes some, though not all, cases of Alzheimer's disease.

Deoxyribonucleic acid, commonly known as DNA, is the basic genetic component. DNA occurs as a double-stranded helix in the nucleus of the cell. Approximately 10,000 DNA pairs compose a gene. A number of genes together, sequenced in a certain order, make up the genetic code. It is this coded information that determines, to a large extent, how each cell develops and behaves, and what products it will make. If just one gene is missing or flawed, a genetic defect in the form of a disease can result.

The largest genetic structure in the cell is the chromosome, which is made up of long strands of DNA chains. Every human cell contains 46 chromosomes: 23 inherited from the mother and 23 inherited from the father. It is through this remarkable organization that individuals inherit their unique physical and intellectual qualities. It is also how individuals may inherit a predisposition to certain diseases, perhaps even Parkinson's disease.

To determine whether PD, or any other disease for that matter, is hereditary, scientists often examine the occurrence of a disease in identical twins. Because identical twins have exactly the same genetic makeup, if one twin inherits a disorder, then it follows that the other twin would be almost certain to inherit it as well. In the case of Parkinson's disease, however, no such coincidence has occurred. In one well-known study, for instance, none of 19 identical twins had PD, while 1 of 43 fraternal (not genetically identical) twins had PD. While this suggests that PD is not an inherited disorder, recent advances in molecular genetics indicate that such a conclusion is simplistic.

New studies and research have added other elements. Several research groups studied the activity of an enzyme called complex I in patients with Parkinson's disease. Complex I plays a central role in the body's capturing of energy from the food we eat and making it available for many other functions. It also helps protect cells from being broken down by certain other enzymes, like those that break down dopamine in the brain. In those patients with PD, however, the functioning of complex I was found to be impaired.

Adding weight to this theory is the fact that MPTP, discussed previously, also blocks the normal functioning of complex I, thus causing the same biochemical defect in MPTP parkinsonians as those with idiopathic PD. Could an inherited lack of some complex I enzyme be related to Parkinson's disease? Although the research on complex I is still in its early stages, it has raised some intriguing questions.

Although a direct and invariable genetic link may never be found to explain Parkinson's disease, the science of genetics will undoubtedly play an increasingly large role in the research and treatment of PD. As you'll learn in the last chapter of this book, scientists have been able to clone healthy substantia nigra cells in the laboratory. In the distant future, replacing dying brain cells with genetically engineered healthy cells may prove to be an effective treatment for PD and other degenerative diseases.

Considering how many parents with PD produce children who never develop the disease, it is clear that even if a tendency to develop Parkinson's disease can be inherited, most people who inherit the "bad" gene will not develop PD. Other factors, most scientists agree, must come into play.

Environmental Causes

Exposure to toxic agents, such as pesticides or industrial chemicals, is another possible explanation for Parkinson's disease. Medical historians have noted that James Parkinson first wrote about the disease at the start of the Industrial Revolution, when environmental pollutants were first introduced. Further, the fact that some parkinsonian patients had inherited inabilities to metabolize certain chemicals, such as manganese or copper, led researchers to look at whether *overdoses* of the same or other chemicals might cause idiopathic Parkinson's disease.

The chemical MPTP, as noted previously, certainly added weight to the theory that a toxic agent could selectively kill substantia nigra cells. In fact, many pesticides and herbicides, such as paraquat, are structurally related to MPP +, the toxic by-product of MPTP. A series of environmental studies conducted in Canada demonstrated that people living in certain areas in the provinces of Saskatchewan and Quebec had a higher rate of PD than the national average. These rural communities were heavily involved in agriculture and in the pulp and paper industries, both of which use large quantities of pesticides and fungicides. Despite an intense investigation, however, no direct involvement of pesticides or fungicides could be linked to the brain damage in Parkinson's disease. Furthermore, other rural areas just as involved in these industries showed no increased rate of Parkinson's disease.

There are several other problems with the environmental exposure hypothesis of PD. First of all, even though the general level of environmental toxins increased dramatically between 1945 and 1979, most studies show no similar dramatic increase in the incidence of PD. Another difficulty is that it is hard to explain how, when two related individuals live in the same household and work in the same environment—and are thus exposed to the same toxins—only one will develop PD.

The most likely explanation, many scientists now think, is that a combination of an as yet unidentified genetic susceptibility *and* exposure to a toxic agent or a virus causes idiopathic PD. In fact, just as there are different causes for meningitis or pneumonia, for instance, there may be several different causes for Parkinson's disease. Patients like Alan who experience depression and other affective disorders in addition to their motor symptoms may be suffering from a different form of Parkinson's disease than, say, Beth who, at least so far, has only experienced problems related to movement.

In addition, some have claimed that the varying rate of progression of Parkinson's disease indicates that different factors or combinations of factors cause PD in different individuals. Indeed, few cases of Parkinson's disease progress in the same way or at the same rate.

Stages of Progression

One of the first questions patients ask concerns the severity of their disease: How bad is my condition now and how bad will it become? Not long ago, as Beth recounted in Chapter One, a diagnosis of Parkinson's disease meant certain and often rapid incapacitation. Today that's no longer true. As stressed throughout this book, with current drug therapy most patients can look forward to many years of active living.

On the other hand, there is no doubt that Parkinson's disease remains an incurable and progressive brain disorder. The symptoms will inevitably worsen over time, even if the patient takes selegiline. How much worse and in what amount of time differ in each individual stricken with the disease.

In fact, many patients find that its very unpredictability is one of the most frustrating things about Parkinson's disease: doctors simply cannot tell how fast or how far the disease will progress. On the other hand, some patients find this aspect of PD a relief: because the course of the disease is unknown, they feel they have more control over the process than they might with more predictable diseases.

Although there is no way to tell what will happen in the future, there are well-accepted methods of rating the disease. These scales not only help assess a patient's "place" in the PD world, they also assist physicians in deciding a course of treatment. It is important to understand that these scales are only indicative of certain standards; they are somewhat subjective and do not necessarily give a complete picture of a patient's condition.

For instance, if you're like most patients, you lived with your disease for some months before receiving your diagnosis. You may be especially nervous and tense when you go to see your doctor, thereby exacerbating your condition. "My tremor is ten times worse when I get nervous," admits Greg, a 60-year-old salesman who has had PD for about six years. "And I've always hated being in hospitals or at the doctor's office."

On the other hand, other patients seem to be at their "best" when they visit their physician and claim that the way they function there is not a good indication of their overall daily performance. Unless you tell him or her, your doctor will not know that you lose your balance when reaching for something on your closet shelf, for instance, or have difficulty unbuttoning your shirt as you undress for bed.

Most physicians familiar with PD, however, are aware of both problems and are not likely to base their decisions regarding treatment solely on one office visit. Eventually, however, he or she will probably use one of the many scales devised to rate PD patients. Among them are the Unified Parkinson's Disease Rating Scale, the Webster Scale, the Hoehn-Yahr Scale, and the Schwab Scale.

The differences among the scales relate to which symptoms are evaluated and the value given to them. In the Hoehn-Yahr Scale, the disease is divided into five stages:

Stage 0 no visible disease
Stage 1 disease involves one side of the body
Stage 2 disease involves both sides of the body, but does not impair balance
Stage 3 disease impairs balance or walking
Stage 4 disease markedly impairs balance or walking
Stage 5 disease results in complete immobility

Needless to say, the areas between each stage of this unpredictable disease are gray, and the amount of time that each patient spends in each stage without progressing to the next varies considerably.

Some physicians use another scale—either alone or in conjunction with the Hoehn-Yahr Scale—that assesses a patient's ability to perform activities of daily living. Some of these scales assign weighted values to particular activities, such as walking, eating, dressing, hygiene, and speaking, and then grade the patient's degree of disability at the time of examination.

It is important to stress that PD involves the *gradual* death of substantia nigra cells, and most patients continue to work and play with only minimal disability for quite some time. Most stages last many years. With the development of better drugs and an understanding of how to manipulate drug therapy (covered in Chapter Four), Parkinson's disease is no longer the dire diagnosis it was just a few years ago.

Nevertheless, you may be feeling anxious and afraid when you receive a diagnosis of PD from your doctor. The next chapter will show you how drug therapy can help you manage your disease. Then, in Chapter Five, you'll learn how to work through the emotional distress you may be feeling and how to devise a healthy, workable strategy to live with your disease in the best way possible.

Chapter Four

Understanding Drug Therapy

SINCE THE time of his diagnosis at the age of 61, Caspar, a 76-year-old retired auto factory worker, has been prescribed about six different kinds of medication and has experienced countless adjustments and readjustments of his drug regimen. Today, fifteen years later, he takes less medication than at any time since the very beginning of his treatment. Although his disease has progressed to the point where he needs almost full-time nursing care, his mind is still sharp, he has hobbies that he enjoys, and, thanks to careful medication adjustment, he is fairly free of serious side effects.

Caspar feels that his journey along the road of Parkinson's disease has been long and hard, but endlessly fascinating. Every day, it seems, he was faced with new problems and found new ways to meet them. He felt, perhaps for the first time, the depth and power of his own optimism and zest for life. He also learned a great deal about drugs—more than he ever thought he'd need to know—and the way they would help him manage his illness. Working together with his physician, Caspar was able to map out a treatment plan that has kept him relatively healthy and satisfied, despite his increasingly disabling illness.

If you have Parkinson's disease, taking drugs of one kind or another will become—if it hasn't already—an integral part of your day-to-day life. Because the course and treatment of PD are such a variable undertaking, it is essential that you, as a PD patient, take an active role in your own therapy.

Less Is Best: The Key to PD Drug Therapy

The single most important rule of successful PD drug therapy is "Less is best." As you'll soon learn, the drugs used to treat PD are powerful. They will help alleviate the symptoms of the disease quite well for a period of time, but at a price. First, they sometimes cause side effects as troubling as the PD symptoms they are meant to relieve. These side effects range from involuntary movements and cramping to mental changes including hallucinations and confusion. Unfortunately, almost every patient, at one time or another in the course of treatment, will experience some drug side effects.

Second, your body may build up a tolerance to these drugs over time, forcing you to take more to receive any benefit. The more drugs you take, of course, the more side effects may result. Another possibility of long-term drug therapy is that your body may develop a sensitivity to the drugs, causing side effects with even the smallest of doses. Balancing benefits and side effects often becomes the greatest challenge of PD treatment.

Just as every patient experiences different symptoms at different stages of the disease, so too do patients react differently to the drugs used to treat them. Alan, with his depression and tremor, may require a different combination of drugs, in different amounts, than Beth, whose symptoms center around rigidity and bradykinesia. To add to the challenge, Alan, who is 6 feet 1 and 200 pounds, may be able to tolerate *less* medicine than Beth, who is 5 feet 3 and 130 pounds. These variables make drug treatment for Parkinson's disease a delicate and often unpredictable process.

Finally, it is essential that you remember that anti-Parkinson drugs, with the possible exception of selegiline, only *mask* symptoms of the disease, they do not attack the underlying pathology. Although your tremor may be lessened and your mobility improved, the dopamine-producing substantia nigra cells in your brain will continue to die. This fact means two things: One, although the drugs are very effective, you may never feel completely well again. Two, eventually—and it may be in 5 years or 25 years—the disease will progress to the point where drug therapy has less effect.

"Not being much of a pill-taker," recalls Caspar, "I decided to learn as much as I could about the drugs I would need to take for my Parkinson's. I read everything I could get my hands on so that when things started to get complicated, what with the side effects and all, I kind of knew what to expect."

Keeping "less is best" in mind, a first step in your role as an involved Parkinson's disease patient or caregiver is to learn about the drugs themselves and how they work. They are your keys to remaining healthy and active for as long as possible.

The Four Classes of Drugs

Generally speaking, there are four different classes of drugs used to alleviate Parkinson's disease symptoms. They each work on a different part of the complex neurotransmission system in the basal ganglia. Their goal: to produce the synapses necessary for proper human movement.

- Anticholinergic therapy: As you may remember from Chapter Two, acetylcholine is another neurotransmitter affected by Parkinson's disease. When dopamine is depleted, the excitatory effect of acetylcholine increases, causing tremor and rigidity. Drugs used to block the action of acetylcholine are called anticholinergics.
- Replacement therapy: The simplest and most direct way of treating the loss of dopamine once produced by substantia nigra cells is to replace it with dopamine from another source. The drug levodopa is converted in the brain to dopamine, replacing the dopamine once produced within the substantia nigra. Levodopa is now given in combination with carbidopa, a substance that blocks the conversion of levodopa outside the brain. This drug combination is called Sinemet. Today, virtually all patients with Parkinson's disease will eventually take the drug Sinemet.
- Dopamine agonists: Once dopamine is released from one neuron, it activates the next neuron by stimulating dopamine receptors arranged on the neuron. Dopamine agonists directly stimulate dendrite receptors, by-passing the need for dopamine itself.

• MAO B inhibitors: These drugs work to make the most of the dopamine your brain is still producing. As you may remember from Chapter Two, dopamine is broken down by an enzyme called monoamine oxidase, or MAO for short. MAO exists both outside and inside the brain; inside the brain, it is known as MAO B. Today, a drug called selegiline (or Eldepryl) has been developed to inhibit the action of MAO B, therefore increasing the amount of dopamine in the nigrostriatal pathway. More important, by blocking MAO B, this drug may slow the progression of PD.

Drugs from among these four classes, separately or in combination with one another, are used to treat the symptoms of Parkinson's disease. All anti-Parkinson drugs have two things in common: First, they are all relatively short-acting drugs. It is unlikely that you'll be able to simply take one pill in the morning and feel relief from your symptoms all day. Even if you need very little medicine, you'll most likely have to space it out in three or four small doses throughout the day. This is especially true for Sinemet.

Second, to repeat an important point: These drugs all work on the brain's complex chemistry. Adding or withdrawing these drugs should be approached with caution. Along with "Less is best," then, is another important adage: "Start low, go slow." Your physician should start you on low doses of medication and gradually increase the amount as needed. Never alter your dosages of medication without first consulting your physician.

In Table 1, you'll find a listing of all the major anti-Parkinson drugs, their effects and side effects, and their most common dosages. If you have specific questions about the drugs you are currently taking, please consult this table and your physician. In Chapter Seven, we'll discuss other drugs, including antidepressants, laxatives, sleeping pills, and over-the-counter medications that may be added to the drug regimen to further relieve PD's symptoms or drug side effects.

Following is a brief overview of anti-Parkinson medications, how they work, and their main side effects.

TABLE 1.
MEDICATIONS COMMONLY USED TO TREAT PARKINSON'S DISEASE

DOPAMINERGICS
Drugs used to replace or mimic the actions of dopamine.

SINEMET

Qualities:	Helps all symptoms. Primary anti-Parkinson drug. Consists of a combination of levodopa and carbidopa. Carbidopa allows levodopa to enter the brain, where it is converted to levodopa.
Dosages:	Expressed as fractions, with top number referring to amount of carbidopa and the bottom number levodopa, in milligrams. Common dosages are 10/100, 25/100, 25/250.
Range of daily dosage:	75–150 mg carbidopa; 75–1,000 mg levodopa.
Side effects:	Nausea, daytime sleepiness, orthostatic hypotension, involuntary movements, decreased appetite, insomnia, cramping. In susceptible patients, it may cause hallucinations, confusion, "on-off" effect.
Special considerations:	Sinemet should be taken one hour before meals for maximum benefit. Should be taken with a whole glass of water or juice. Crackers should be taken if Sinemet causes stomach upset.

SINEMET CR

Qualities:	A controlled-release form of Sinemet.
Dosage:	50/200.
Range of daily dosage:	75–200 mg carbidopa; 200–1,000 mg levodopa.
Side effects:	Same side effects as with regular Sinemet.
Special considerations:	May be especially useful in patients with "on-off" effects.

ANTICHOLINERGICS
Anticholinergics block the action of the neurotransmitter aceytlcholine, helping to regain balance between acetylcholine and dopamine. Effective against rigidity and tremor, not against bradykinesia or akinesia. May be used alone early in treatment, or with Sinemet. Poor response or side effects with one anticholinergic does not exclude a trial with another.

ARTANE

Chemical name:	Trihexyphenidyl HCL.
Qualities:	Reduces tremor, drooling, and rigidity. This medication, like Cogentin, is a synthetic antispasmodic drug which has a relaxing effect on smooth muscle.
Dosages:	Tablets of 2 mg, 5 mg, and long-acting 5 mg.
Range of daily dosage:	2–15 mg.
Side effects:	Similar to Cogentin.
Special considerations:	Report side effects.

COGENTIN

Chemical name:	Benzotropine mesylate.
Qualities:	Reduces tremor, rigidity, and drooling.
Dosages:	0.5 mg, 1 mg, 2 mg.
Range of daily dosage:	0.5–6 mg.
Side effects:	Dry mouth, nausea, vomiting, confusion, difficulty swallowing or speaking, blurred vision, loss of appetite and/or weight, depression, hallucinations, constipation, urinary retention. Can worsen glaucoma.
Special considerations:	Use cautiously in elderly patients and patients with a history of confusion. Use cautiously in men with enlarged prostate gland.

DOPAMINE AGONISTS

Mimic the effects of dopamine by directly stimulating the dopamine receptors. Most commonly used early in combination with Sinemet. Agonists may also be started when patients are no longer responding to Sinemet satisfactorily. Agonists may smooth out the fluctuating effect (wearing off) or "on-off" often seen in Parkinson's patients on chronic levodopa treatment. They are started at low doses and built up gradually over several weeks before therapeutic results are achieved. If dyskinsias increase, then a reduction in levodopa is indicated.

PARLODEL

Chemical name:	Bromocriptine mesylate.
Qualities:	Helps all aspects of Parkinson's disease. Used in combination with Sinemet to reduce symptoms and ameliorate severity of adverse reactions associated with long-term levodopa therapy,

especially dyskinsias, wearing off and "on-off." Acts directly on the D2 receptors.

Dosages: Tablet, 2.5 mg; capsule, 5 mg.
Range of daily dosage: 1.25–30 mg.
Side effects: Orthostatic hypotension, nausea, blurred vision, hallucinations.
Special considerations: May take several weeks for an effect to occur.

PERMAX

Chemical name: Pergolide mesylate.
Qualities: Helps all aspects. Acts on both D1 and D2 receptors. Used in combination with Sinemet to reduce symptoms, may allow reduction in amount of Sinemet.
Dosages: Tablets 0.05 mg, 0.25 mg, 1 mg.
Range of daily dosage: 0.05–5 mg.
Side effects: Similar to bromocriptine (Parlodel).
Special considerations: Similar to bromocriptine (Parlodel). May be effective in some patients who are no longer responding to bromocriptine.

OTHER MEDICATIONS

SYMMETREL

Chemical name: Amantadine.
Qualities: An antiviral compound; it relieves tremors, rigidity, and bradykinesia.
Dosage: 100 mg capsules.
Range of daily dosage: 100–300 mg.
Side effects: Swelling of the feet, loss of appetite, dizziness, anxiety, depression, hallucinations, urinary retention, blotchy legs, insomnia.
Special considerations: Should be used carefully in elderly patients.

DEPRENYL (ELDEPRYL, SELEGILINE)

Qualities: An MAO B inhibitor. Increases effect of dopamine by blocking the enzyme MAO B that normally breaks down dopamine. Leads to increase in amount of dopamine in brain.

Usually used in conjunction with Sinemet. Although not officially approved for this specific use, there is a large body of evidence that strongly suggests that deprenyl may slow progression of PD.

Dosage: Capsule, 5 mg.
Range of daily dosage: 10 mg.
Side effects: Loss of appetite, nausea, dizziness, anxiety, insomnia. In susceptible individuals it may cause confusion, hallucinations.

INDERAL

Chemical name: Propranolol.
Qualities: May reduce tremors.
Side effects: Lightheadedness, insomnia, weakness, depression, fatigue. In men it may cause impotence.

FLUORINEF

Qualities: Used to raise blood pressure by retaining salt.
Dosage: 0.1–0.5 mg.
Side effects: Leg swelling, hypertension.

Would You Believe Belladonna? Anticholinergic Therapy

The progress of medical research and treatment often depends on a combination of chance and keen observation. In the nineteenth century, for instance, French neurologist Jean-Martin Charcot, studying the newly defined Parkinson's disease, found that when his PD patients took certain drugs to treat unrelated stomach disorders, their PD symptoms also improved dramatically. The drugs they used were plant extracts, or "tinctures." He and his associates then began to treat their PD patients with similar drugs.

One of these tinctures was extracted from belladonna, a plant of the deadly nightshade family. As ominous as the nightshade family sounds, however, it has provided medical science with many useful medications. For nearly 100 years, drugs derived from these plants represented the only treatment for Parkinson's disease.

Belladonna, scientists later discovered, contains two active in-

TABLE 2.
Drugs Contraindicated in PD Patients

The term "contraindicated" means that the drug should not be given. Many of the drugs affect the dopamine system and may bring out latent symptoms or increase symptoms that are already present. All symptoms usually disappear after the drugs are stopped.

Drug Category	Trade Name	Generic Name
Antipsychotic	Haldol	Haloperidol
	Trilafon	Perphenazine
	Thorazine	Chlorpromazine
	Stelazine	Trifluoperazine
	Prolixin, Permitil	Flufenazine
	Navane	Thiothixene
	Mellaril	Thioridazine
Antidepressant	Triavil	Combination of perphenazine and amitriptyline
	Nardil	Phenelzine
	Parnate	Tranylcypromine
Antivomiting	Compazine	Prochlorperazine
	Reglan	Metoclopramide
	Torecan	Thiethylperazine
Miscellaneous	Serpasil	Reserpine
	Aldomet	Alpha-methyldopa

gredients: hyoscine (or scopolamine) and atropine. Both of these substances work to relax smooth muscle and reduce secretions in the bronchial tubes, salivary glands, stomach, and intestinal organs. They do so by blocking acetylcholine, the chemical transmitter that would otherwise activate these organs. Extracts of the belladonna plant are, then, anticholinergics.

Once the chemical structures of acetylcholine and its blocking agents were understood, scientists developed synthetic (man-made) drugs that were more effective than the natural drugs derived from plants. Artane, Cogentin, and Kemadrin are just a few of the most common brand names of the anticholinergics available specifically to treat Parkinson's disease and other parkinsonian conditions.

Related to these are antihistamines, most often used to treat allergies and cold symptoms. The major effect of these drugs is to block the action of histamine, which is formed in the body during allergic reactions. In addition, antihistamines also have anticholinergic effects.

Like many anti-Parkinson drugs, anticholinergics may cause a number of annoying side effects. Because they act to reduce glandular secretions, dry mouth often results from taking anticholinergics. A decrease in the actions of smooth muscles in the eye, throat, and intestines may cause blurry vision, dizziness, difficulty in swallowing, constipation, and urinary retention.

Anticholinergics may also disturb mental function. Anyone who has taken an antihistamine for a cold or allergy is sure to have noted its warning about not driving or operating heavy machinery. Drowsiness, dizziness, and slight confusion may result from even small doses taken over a short period of time. With the long-term use associated with Parkinson's disease, some patients will experience more severe effects, including hallucinations, confusion, depression, listlessness.

Based on patient observation, physicians estimate that about 50 percent of PD patients will benefit to some degree from anticholinergic drugs. They are especially effective in treating mild cases of PD and often are among the first drugs prescribed to a newly diagnosed patient. Many patients are treated with anticholinergics for a number of months or years, staving off the need for other medication for as long as possible. Because they have a relaxing effect on smooth muscle, anticholinergics are especially helpful in reducing tremor, but are usually not effective against bradykinesia, walking, or balance problems. As these problems increase in the course of the disease, levodopa therapy is necessary. Anticholinergics may also be used in conjunction with levodopa in later stages of the disease.

An Antiviral Solution: Amantadine

Another drug commonly prescribed early in PD treatment is amantadine, also known as Symmetrel. An antiviral medication long used to prevent the development of flu, amantadine, like anti-cholinergic therapy, was discovered to have anti-Parkinson effects quite by accident. A parkinsonian patient, taking Symmetrel for a flu, reported to her physician that her PD symptoms improved while she was taking the drug. Further research confirmed this observation and amantadine became a common antiparkinsonian drug in the late 1960s.

Exactly how amantadine works on the parkinsonian brain remains unclear. It appears to help release dopamine from within the remaining substantia nigra cells, thereby stimulating the activity of the striatum. Unfortunately, amantadine also causes side effects, ranging from swelling of the feet and ankles to a purplish skin mottling of the legs to visual hallucinations and mental confusion.

Nevertheless, for many mild cases of Parkinson's disease, Symmetrel works quite well to reduce symptoms, including tremor, rigidity, and bradykinesia. Like anticholinergic therapy, treatment with Symmetrel may often delay for several months or more the need for levodopa therapy. It may also be used in conjunction with other anti-Parkinson drugs as the disease progresses.

The Miracle of Levodopa

As early as the 1950s, scientists suspected that a lack of dopamine in the striatum caused Parkinson's disease. Unfortunately, they did not yet have the key to replacing this crucial chemical in the brain.

Their first obstacle was the brain itself. Considering its complicated chemistry, it is no wonder that the brain is protected from unwanted substances that might disturb its delicate equilibrium. A thin membrane of tissue, called the blood-brain barrier, separates the blood from brain cells. This membrane is semipermeable; certain substances can pass through, while others cannot. Dopamine, for instance, is unable to cross the blood-brain barrier. Therefore, although dopamine can be administered orally or intravenously, it cannot reach the brain.

Levodopa, dopamine's precursor, on the other hand, can pass through the blood-brain barrier. As you may remember from Chapter Two, levodopa is converted to dopamine in the brain by the enzyme dopa decarboxylase. Levodopa was initially used by W. Birkenmayer in Vienna in 1960, who injected it into patients with Parkinson's disease. Although many patients initially improved dramatically, the effects were brief and most patients experienced profound nausea, vomiting, and hypotension (lowered blood pressure). Most physicians concluded that although levodopa was a promising drug, it was not a practical treatment for Parkinson's disease. Some physicians then attempted to give levodopa by mouth, but because even low doses produced nausea and vomiting, the trials were discontinued.

In 1967, G. Cotzias reintroduced levodopa as a treatment for PD. Cotzias had achieved remarkable success with levodopa in treating Chilean manganese miners who had developed a form of parkinsonism related to manganese poisoning. Cotzias reasoned that levodopa could be given to PD patients if the starting dose was low and built up gradually. His work with levodopa in seemingly end-stage PD patients revolutionized the treatment of PD.

Anyone who has read *Awakenings*, the remarkable book by Dr. Oliver Sacks, or seen the movie based upon it, will remember the excitement and then tragedy that levodopa often caused. During the late 1960s, postencephalitic parkinsonians, some of them with very severe symptoms, were given large doses of levodopa. Miraculously, many of these patients were able to move about for the first time in 20 years or more. Released from states of immobility, they were able to stand straight and tall, walk and dance, smile, and look at the world around them.

Unfortunately, in these patients, levodopa was not the miracle drug it first appeared to be. Less than 10 percent of the levodopa dose was actually getting into the brain; a full 90 percent was converted to dopamine in the body. The dopamine generated in the body caused many patients to experience prolonged bouts of nausea and vomiting—not because dopamine affected the digestive tract but because it provoked the vomiting center located at the base of the brain, outside the blood-brain barrier. In fact, until physicians more thoroughly understood the principles of levodopa therapy, vomiting was one of the only signs physicians had that their patients were being overdosed on this powerful chemical.

These large dosages of levodopa given to postencephalitic patients caused other severe side effects, including hallucinations, involuntary movements (dyskinesias), and emotional crises (depression and mania). Furthermore, patients soon built up either a tolerance to the drug or a sensitivity to it. In either case, the therapeutic value of levodopa diminished quickly and patients were once again overwhelmed by the effects of parkinsonism.

One more step was needed before levodopa could be considered a successful therapy for Parkinson's disease. In the mid-1970s, another drug was developed that blocked the conversion of levodopa outside the brain, allowing about 80 percent of the levodopa to be converted to dopamine in the striatum. Called carbidopa, this inhibitor cannot pass through the blood-brain barrier and, therefore, does not affect the conversion process inside the brain. In the United States, the drug composed of a combination of carbidopa and levodopa is known as Sinemet.

Sinemet is available in three different dosage forms: 10 mg of carbidopa to 100 mg of levodopa (10/100); 25 mg of carbidopa to 250 mg of levodopa (25/250); and 25 mg of carbidopa to 100 mg of levodopa (25/100). As a rule, most patients below the age of 70 require 75 to 100 mg of carbidopa for the levodopa to be most effective. Above the age of 70, patients often require much less carbidopa.

Today, Sinemet is the single most effective drug available to treat the symptoms of Parkinson's disease. Indeed, most patients manage to control their symptoms for many years, with relatively few side effects, by taking Sinemet every day. Nevertheless, the fact that levodopa remains the active ingredient means that the same kinds of problems experienced with pure levodopa will also occur with Sinemet over a longer period of time.

Like levodopa alone, Sinemet eventually loses some of its effectiveness. About 50 percent of all PD patients find that, after about three to five years, the effects of Sinemet decrease. Their parkinsonian symptoms worsen, and more medication is needed to achieve the same mobility and function that lower dosages achieved in the past. After ten years, the percentage of patients claiming a decrease in function climbs to 80 percent.

During the earlier stages of the disease, the benefits of one dose of Sinemet often last until the next dose takes effect. The symptoms of Parkinson's disease, then, are successfully masked evenly throughout the day. As time passes, however, one dose no longer lasts until the next one "kicks in," so to speak. A drop in mobility and/or an increase in tremor occurs between doses. Some patients compare this "on-off" phenomenon to a light switch: When they're "on," their symptoms are masked and their function is improved. When they're "off," all symptoms are severe. In advanced cases of PD, patients who exhibit this "on-off" phenomenon may go from being wheelchair-bound and immobile to being fully ambulatory within just a few minutes after the drug kicks in.

A new form of Sinemet may help to alleviate some of these problems. This drug, which will be in a tablet composed of 50 mg of carbidopa and 200 mg of levodopa, is designed in a *controlled-release* formula or Sinemet CR. Sinemet CR does not produce as large a peak level as regular Sinemet, but the effects last about twice as long. This longer-acting drug may accomplish two things in some patients: it may help to smooth out the "on-off" periods and reduce the number of times patients need to take Sinemet during the day. Therefore it is particularly indicated in patients with wearing-"off" phenomenon.

Both Sinemet and the new Sinemet CR cause some side effects similar to those caused by anticholinergics and amantadine: dry mouth, constipation, nausea, mental confusion, and depression. In addition, Sinemet may produce dyskinesias, or involuntary movements. Ironically, dyskinesias are caused by an *overdose* of dopamine in the brain. In effect, the striatum is overloaded by the neurotransmitter, thereby creating too much movement. These involuntary movements may involve any part of the body and include head bobbing, lip smacking, tongue thrusting, leg writhing, hand clasping, and trunk twisting. Dyskinesia is related, almost always, to how much Sinemet a patient has been taking and for how long. The more Sinemet you take, and the longer you take it, the more likely it is that dyskinesias will become a problem for you.

Pushing the Right Buttons: The Dopamine Agonists

During the 1950s, a new class of drugs was studied. Instead of replacing dopamine in the brain, these drugs *mimicked* the action of dopamine. In other words, they directly stimulated dopamine receptors in the striatum, bypassing the need for dopamine itself.

Interestingly enough, the first dopamine agonist used, apomorphine, was an emetic; it acted on the same vomiting center that would later be affected by levodopa therapy.

The early dopamine agonists were too toxic to provide sustained and reliable relief from PD symptoms. About a decade later, however, a synthetic drug used to treat certain endocrine problems in women was shown to have dopamine-agonist capabilities, but without causing severe side effects. Known as bromocriptine, or Parlodel, this drug was found to stimulate the striatal receptors known as D2 receptors. It was first used as an anti-Parkinson agent by D. Calne and then, later, A. Lieberman.

Dopamine agonists, although not as potent as levodopa, have certain advantages. Agonists do not have to be converted in the brain to be effective, they can be given in small amounts, and they may improve symptoms not improved by levodopa. Moreover, because agonists decrease the requirement for levodopa, less dopamine accumulates and there may be fewer side effects such as dyskinesias. In fact, increasing evidence supports using agonists earlier, before fluctuations or dyskinesias start.

While many agonists have been developed, only three are widely used: bromocriptine (Parlodel), lisuride (Dopergin), and a relatively new drug, pergolide (Permax), introduced by A. Lieberman. Most often used in combination with Sinemet, bromocriptine and lisuride are usually prescribed to moderate or advanced patients who have begun to experience the "on-off" effect associated with long-term levodopa therapy. Bromocriptine often gives enough of a "push" to the dopamine-hungry striatal receptors that the patient no longer shuts off before his or her next dose of Sinemet kicks in. Adding Parlodel may also allow for a considerable reduction in the amount of levodopa taken by the patient, which may decrease troubling side effects and prolong the drug's effectiveness.

Unlike bromocriptine, which stimulates only D2 receptors, pergolide stimulates both D1 and D2 receptors. Pergolide is added to a patient's drug regimen, again, usually in combination with Sinemet. Some patients respond better to bromocriptine, others to pergolide.

Dopamine agonists, too, can cause side effects, including dizziness, nausea, hallucinations, diarrhea, and constipation. Dyskinesias may occur with the addition of a dopamine agonist, indicating that, together with the effects of Sinemet, the striatal receptors are receiving too much stimulation. Several careful adjustments in medication often must be made.

Making the Most of What You've Got: Selegiline

During the early 1960s, scientists discovered a group of drugs that could block MAO, the enzyme responsible for breaking down excess chemical transmitters, both in the brain and in the body. These MAO inhibitors were developed to treat depression, then believed to be caused by a lack of dopamine in the cerebral cortex.

Scientists studying Parkinson's disease were as excited about MAO inhibitors as the psychiatrists treating depression. If these drugs could increase the amount of dopamine in one part of the brain, then they might be able to increase the supply in the striatum as well. Unfortunately, most of the early MAO inhibitors not only inhibited the breakdown of dopamine in the brain but also acted in the liver, causing damage to that organ. This resulted in the escape of a compound called tyramine, found in some foods such as cheese, into the blood stream. Tyramine can, in some patients, elevate blood pressure markedly and result in stroke.

One drug, however, was developed by a company in Hungary and studied by Joseph Knoll at the University of Budapest in the early 1960s. The drug was called selegiline and it did not appear to inhibit the breakdown of dopamine anywhere except in the striatum. Indeed, scientists would later prove that selegiline is MAO B selective; it affects only enzymatic activity in the brain.

Because of Knoll's insistence that selegiline did not have toxic effects, W. Birkenmayer used the drug on his PD patients. He studied the drug's effects for several years, finding that, on the average, those taking a combination of levodopa and selegiline remained active and mobile about a year longer than those taking levodopa alone. After Birkenmayer released his remarkable findings, interest in MAO inhibitors increased when the MPTP story (described in Chapter Three) broke. MPTP is converted by MAO B to another chemical called MPP+, which then destroyed substantia nigra cells. Selegiline, by blocking MAO B, halts the production of MPP+, thereby preventing the death of substantia nigra cells.

These findings continue to excite researchers and clinicians involved with Parkinson's disease. Selegiline appears to have two effects: First, it reduces the symptoms of Parkinson's disease by increasing the amount of dopamine available in the striatum. Second, Birkenmayer's observations—and those of others since then—indicate that selegiline may retard the progression of the disease itself. The drug appears to act as a neuroprotector, shielding brain cells from premature degeneration. If so, selegiline could be used to treat a whole range of neurodegenerative diseases, including both Parkinson's and Alzheimer's.

Selegiline (or deprenyl), approved by the FDA in 1989 and marketed under the brand name Eldepryl, is being prescribed by doctors across the country to treat both newly diagnosed and more-advanced cases. It has side effects similar to those experienced with levodopa and is prescribed alone and in combination with Sinemet. As it now appears selegiline has a protective effect, physicians hope that it will extend the length of time a patient can function both before and after requiring levodopa therapy. For moderate to advanced cases, selegiline appears to increase the amount of dopamine in the striatum, thereby giving an often much-needed "boost" to the effects of Sinemet.

A Word About "Drug Holidays"

There is some evidence that patients who have been taking levodopa for a number of years may benefit from a period of withdrawal from Sinemet, especially when they are experiencing severe side effects. Nicknamed "levodopa drug holidays," these drug-free periods usually last 10 to 14 days and are meant to "rest" the brain's overtaxed dopamine receptors. They must take place within a hospital setting, as patients with advanced disease will lose most of their mobility and will need constant care.

During the 1970s and 1980s, drug holidays were fairly common. However, many doctors now feel that the benefits of drug withdrawal are not worth either the medical risks—including pneumonia—or the psychological agony experienced by most patients.

Instead, most physicians believe that more frequent and careful medication adjustments will minimize the side effects of levodopa and maximize benefits without the need for debilitating, and expensive, hospital stays. An exception to this general rule is in cases of severe levodopa overdose.

The Puzzle: Managing Parkinson's Disease with Drug Therapy

At what point should I start levodopa therapy? How much is too much Sinemet? Is there something that will make my tremor stop without causing me to hallucinate? How long will drug therapy allow me to keep my job?

Whether you've just been diagnosed with Parkinson's disease or you've suffered with the disease for a number of years, you're bound to have questions about what approach to drug therapy is right to you. Unfortunately, even your physician can give you no more than a best guess as to what drugs will work for you and for how long.

As has been stated often in this book, every patient experiences Parkinson's disease in a different way. The course of your disease and your reactions to the drugs used to treat your particular set of symptoms are unique. If you've recently been diagnosed, you may be asking yourself if you need to take selegiline. Again, that's a question only you and your physician can answer together. Consider the following few cases of recently diagnosed Parkinson's disease patients:

- Mark, a 55-year-old worker in a meat-packing plant, is anxious to keep his job—and his medical insurance—but finds that rigidity and tremor get in the way.
- Jessie, a 75-year-old retired lawyer who is an avid gardener and walker, wants to keep as active as possible for as long as possible. Her symptoms are moderate, with balance problems and lingering depression troubling her the most.
- Rosemary, a 33-year-old single woman, works as a salesperson at a department store. Her symptoms are minor: Her right leg drags slightly and she has a mild tremor in her right hand. She feels quite well physically, but has deep fears about the long road ahead.

Most researchers would agree that all these patients should be on selegiline, which may act as a neuroprotector. In addition, each of these patients, placed on strong enough doses of Sinemet, would quickly see most of the symptoms almost completely eradicated—but they might experience side effects. Indeed, all decisions concerning drug treatment for PD must be considered in light of the long-term effects, and drugs must be prescribed on a highly individual basis.

Mark, for instance, is a manual laborer. He needs as much mobility and strength as he can possibly get. Should he be placed on Sinemet, in addition to selegiline, right away? Probably. Will drug therapy allow him to keep his job? In the short term, Mark will probably find that his medication allows him to work at a fairly normal capacity most of the time. But he should start now to think about finding a new job within his company that requires less physical activity. He should not assume that the medicine will continue to work as well as it does at the beginning of therapy or that he can simply move on to higher dosages later.

Jessie, on the other hand, is a different kind of patient. Most important, she is older. Otherwise in very good health, she wants her last years of life to be as active as possible. Therefore, although she too must be careful not to take too much Sinemet, she is old enough that the drug's effectiveness may outlive her. Her doctor may well decide to prescribe whatever dosages of medicine it takes to make her comfortable without causing unpleasant side effects.

Completely different from both Mark and Jessie, Rosemary probably should not take Sinemet right away. She is so young and her symptoms are so mild that treatment with levodopa should be staved off for as long as possible. In fact, she may not need any drug other than selegiline for a number of months, or she may be prescribed low doses of an anticholinergic or Symmetrel for a year or two. Later, she and her doctor, together, will make the decision on when levodopa therapy is needed.

As you can see, drug therapy for Parkinson's disease combines remarkably effective—but toxic—drugs with a trial-and-error approach to dosages and scheduling. You as a patient must consider both the short-term and the long-term view of your disease before deciding, with your physician, what treatment is right for you.

Robert Feldman, professor and chairman of University Hospital's Department of Neurology in Boston, Massachusetts, refers to "targets of therapy" when discussing drug treatment with his patients. As effective as anti-Parkinson drugs are, they will never make you "as good as new." Instead, you will have to accept limits on some aspects of your physical life.

Think carefully about which of your symptoms or side effects bother you most. Can you live with a small tremor if it means you don't need to take as much medicine? Would you rather deal with dry mouth or constipation than suffer with a tremor or rigidity? Are your mornings quiet enough so that you can take less medicine then, but ingest a larger dose in the afternoon when you visit friends or exercise?

Lisa, a 58-year-old mother of two, is a good example. The amount of medicine she needs to alleviate her symptoms now causes troubling side effects. If she takes enough medication to loosen her muscles, she suffers from dyskinesias and hallucinations. If she takes a little less medicine, she experiences a decrease in mobility and an increase in tremor—but her troubling hallucinations and dyskinesias decrease dramatically.

Lisa chose to accept a little less mobility rather than accept the side effects. Her teenage children help with some of the chores that are now more difficult for her to do alone. When she needs a bit more medicine to get through a dinner party or an evening out, her doctor has given her permission to take what is quaintly known as a "Cinderella" pill, an extra dose of Sinemet to boost her performance. This occasional extra dose rarely results in either dyskinesias or hallucinations.

Patients like Lisa, knowledgeable about Parkinson's disease and its symptoms and side effects, can expect to receive the most flexibility and satisfaction from their drug therapy. The following three cases will help you further understand the challenges of Parkinson's disease and its therapy as it progresses over years.

Three Case Histories

Mild

Hugh, the 24-year-old marketing executive whom you met in Chapter One, has a relatively mild case of Parkinson's disease.

Although diagnosed just two years ago, he's pretty sure he's had symptoms since his junior or senior year in high school. As you may remember, Hugh went from neurologist to neurologist before receiving his diagnosis.

Because of the increasing rigidity in his legs and his worsening balance problems, Hugh's doctor felt that, despite his relatively mild disease and his youth, treatment with Sinemet was necessary. Hugh takes three Sinemet tablets a day, each with a strength of 25/100 (which means he's getting a total of 75 milligrams of carbidopa and 300 milligrams of levodopa every day). In addition, his doctor has prescribed the MAO B inhibitor selegiline. Hugh takes two selegiline pills each day, one in the morning and one in the afternoon.

Generally, Hugh takes a half a Sinemet pill soon after he gets up, a whole one about 30 minutes before lunch, a half in the afternoon at about 4:00 or 5:00 and then a whole pill at night, around 8:00 or 9:00. The nighttime pill may seem unusual because, generally, no medication is necessary at night since patients are inactive. However, some patients find that they cannot sleep because they cannot turn around in bed at night unless they take Sinemet.

Hugh, for instance, sleeps better and can get up more easily in the morning by taking Sinemet at night. "I was never a morning person to begin with," he recounts, "and with the stiffness of Parkinson's disease, mornings were a nightmare, so to speak. I find that if I take a Sinemet at night, I at least have an even chance of getting out of bed on time in the morning!"

Over the past several months, Hugh has learned what to expect from his medications and, with his doctor's permission, has begun to experiment with the timing of his pill-taking. For instance, if he knows he has an important client meeting in the afternoon at two o'clock, he may wait to take his pill until after lunch. If he feels especially stiff in the morning and wants to take full advantage of the A.M. to exercise, he may take a whole pill before breakfast.

Never does Hugh take more than the prescribed three 25/100 Sinemets per day. He does, however, feel free to decide how and when to "spend" them, so to speak.

So far, after nearly a year, Hugh still feels no side effects at all from the medications. He leads an active, busy, normal life. He works out two or three times a week at a local gym and bicycles outside, weather permitting, almost every day. He does find that lifting weights can cause a worsening of his tremor; he has had to cut down on the weights but has kept the repetitions the same.

Hugh finds most of his symptoms almost completely alleviated by Sinemet, although he continues to have trouble with his speech. He finds he talks too fast and tends to repeat words or phrases often. He's been seeing a speech therapist once a week. Now that he's had the problem evaluated and has learned some exercises, he'll probably go just once a month or every other month in the future.

Hugh feels confident that he'll be able to outlast his disease, even though he is just 24 years old. So far, he's doing all he can to make that possible. He exercises, takes as little medication as possible, keeps his spirits up, and, most important, stays as informed as possible about the disease.

Moderate

Margaret, the 65-year-old woman whom you met in Chapter One, was diagnosed with Parkinson's disease about five years ago. Like Hugh, she feels that her symptoms predated her diagnosis by at least four years. Margaret retired from her job as a high school English teacher just before being diagnosed, although she still substitute-teaches on occasion. A widow, she recently moved in with her daughter, son-in-law, and two grandchildren.

By the time her physician made the diagnosis of Parkinson's disease, Margaret was at a Stage 2 on the Hoehn-Yahr Scale. Although she feels that she has pretty much held her own since that time, she does admit that her symptoms are getting worse. She has never experienced tremor, but is plagued with rigidity, bradykinesia, and gait disturbances: both festination and freezing.

"It's awful. It seems as if I'm either completely still or absolutely running. When it's really bad, it takes such an effort to pull myself out of my chair I think I'll have to crawl to the kitchen. But I find myself almost running and have to catch at the wall to slow myself down. Then, when I get to the doorway, I freeze. I can't seem to pick up my foot and take the next step. When I really concentrate, I can get myself going again. But one time, I was there for almost five minutes before my daughter came by. She just gave me a little push and I was fine, but, boy, did it frighten me!"

For about eight months following her diagnosis, Margaret took only amantadine. She took three 100 milligram capsules a day, one in the morning, one just before lunch, and one just before dinner. As her symptoms worsened, her doctor decided the time was right to begin levodopa therapy. He started her out on three 10/100 Sinemets a day: one in the morning, one-half at 1:00 P.M., one at 4:00 and one-half at 7:00. At the same time, he slowly withdrew the amantadine.

Over the years, Margaret has slowly increased her dosage of Sinemet. She now takes three 25/250 mg tablets daily on the same schedule. The days that Margaret teaches, which average about twice a month, her doctor has allowed her a "Cinderella" pill in the middle of the day.

"The morning dose used to get me going so well I only needed a half dose before lunch," admits Margaret, "but now I often feel my half dose of Sinemet at one o'clock doesn't get me through an afternoon of teaching. I take a full pill then. Depending on how I'm feeling and what I've got scheduled at night, I may decide to skip the half pill at seven. Usually, however, I simply add the extra half and call it a good day!"

Margaret was recently prescribed two doses a day of selegiline, one in the morning and one in the afternoon. She feels that this really gives her an extra boost of energy, sustaining her through hours that used to be her "down" time. Although Margaret's doctor is skeptical about selegiline's protective capabilities, he is convinced that its symptomatic effects will ease her growing freezing and rigidity problems. "My goal for Margaret, and for all my patients for that matter, is to keep her as active as possible for as long as possible," her doctor remarks. "She loves to teach, she loves to play with her grandchildren, and she loves to read. I see no reason why she can't enjoy doing those things for many more years."

Margaret, who lives just outside Minneapolis, has one other joy: cross-country skiing. "Believe it or not, I've been able to ski at least twice every winter. Parkinson's disease may slow me down a bit, but I'm still a strong old gal."

Advanced

Caspar, the man whom you met at the beginning of the chapter, has now had Parkinson's disease for 15 years. Now at Stage 4 on the Hoehn-Yahr Scale, Caspar is usually wheelchair-bound, although he can stand up and walk with assistance. He requires help to eat, dress, and bathe. Mary, his wife of 35 years, takes care of most of his needs but has recently hired full-time nursing help during the day. His speech volume is low, his words are slurred, and he has trouble swallowing liquids.

Until quite recently, Caspar was taking four 25/250 Sinemets, for a total of 1,000 mg of levodopa, and two doses of 5 mg capsules of bromocriptine every day. In addition, he took two doses of 2 mg tablets of Artane to control his tremor. He took one of each pill at 7:00 A.M., about one-half hour before breakfast; one Sinemet before lunch at 11:30; a Sinemet, a bromocriptine, and an Artane at 3:00; and the last Sinemet at around 6:30, an hour before dinner.

For a time, this schedule worked well for Caspar. He felt "on" most of the day and was able to read and visit with friends, especially during the morning, when he felt the best. The major side effects of his medication, including constipation and occasional lapses in memory, were manageable to him.

About six months ago, however, Caspar began to experience the "on-off" phenomenon more severely. "It used to take about half an hour for the drugs to kick in. Then it was more like an hour, maybe more, before I would feel better. Then, when they did kick in, I'd start having these jerky, writhing movements I couldn't control, though I could get up and move around if Mary or the nurse was there to help me. But then the dose wouldn't last as long as it used to. I'd start to tighten up a good half hour before the next dose was due. Pretty soon I was spending most of the day stuck in a chair, just staring straight ahead. And my tremor never seemed to stop."

Most troubling for Caspar, and for his wife, however, were the mental disturbances that began at about this time. Although Caspar had had some trouble with confusion and disorientation in the past, he now started to hallucinate frequently. "It was nothing terrible, really, just a little weird," Mary recalled. "He'd tell me that there was a dog sleeping in front of the fireplace or people outside in the yard. But when I looked nothing was there. What scared me most, though, was when he started telling me that the nurse was trying to hurt him or poison him. That's when I really got upset."

Caspar appeared to have two contradictory problems: He was not able to get through the day with an even response from the drugs he was taking, the "off" periods were now longer than the "ons." Secondly, he was experiencing symptoms that pointed to an overdose of levodopa: dyskinesias, hallucinations, and paranoia.

It was clear to Caspar's physician that Caspar was taking too much Sinemet, but he needed something to help even out his response. The solution: substitute pergolide for bromocriptine and reduce the amount of Sinemet. The amount of Artane remained the same.

Caspar's daily drug schedule now looked like this:

7:00 A.M.:   one 25/100 Sinemet, one 2 mg Artane, one 0.25 mg Permax
11:30 A.M.:   one 25/100 Sinemet
1:30 P.M.:   one-half 25/100 Sinemet
3:00 P.M.:   one 25/100 Sinemet, one 2 mg Artane, one 0.25 mg Permax
5:00 P.M.:   one-half 25/100 Sinemet
6:30 P.M.:   one 25/100 Sinemet

Instead of taking 1,000 mg of levodopa every day, Caspar now has cut that total in half. His days are much more even for two reasons. First, the addition of pergolide (Permax) gives him the extra "push" his dopamine-hungry striatum needs. Also, Caspar is taking smaller doses of Sinemet, but at shorter intervals during the day. The "extra" half pills he takes at 1:30 and at 5:00 help him through the afternoons—when his symptoms had been at their worst.

Life is getting more and more difficult for Caspar, and for his wife, Mary. In recent months, they have talked with their physician about the possibility of entering Caspar into a full-time elderly-care facility, a difficult decision for this loving couple.

*   *   *

As you can see from just these three case histories, there are many challenges of Parkinson's disease and the side effects of the drugs used to treat it. The A to Z Guide to Symptoms and Side Effects in Chapter Seven will provide you with tips about how to deal with the myriad challenges, both physical and emotional, that face you and your family. Everything from dressing yourself in the morning to dealing with sexual dysfunction to coping with depression will be discussed in this section.

In the meantime, you'll discover in the next chapter how important it is to stay fit and eat right, despite the limits Parkinson's disease may put on your body.

Chapter Five

The Role of Diet and Exercise

IF YOU have Parkinson's disease, keeping fit is nearly as important as taking your medication. The disease you have will eventually make even ordinary movements more difficult to perform. It will take more energy and strength simply to walk to the corner grocery, or braid your hair, or lift yourself out of a chair than it has in the past. It's important, then, that your muscles stay as strong and flexible as possible.

If you're overweight, you'll have even more trouble getting around because you'll be carrying extra cargo. The trimmer you are, the easier it will be to maneuver your body in bed, on a bicycle, or cooking dinner for your family. Moreover, by eating the right kinds of food, you not only will maintain better general health but may also help reduce the symptoms and side effects of PD. Eating high-fiber foods and drinking plenty of water, for instance, will help you control constipation, one of the most annoying side effects of PD and some PD medication. (For more information about relieving constipation, see pages 124–25 in The A to Z Guide in Chapter Seven.)

Although there is no single eating or exercise plan mandatory for parkinsonians, there are specific diets and exercise routines that can be recommended. This chapter provides a general overview of the best way for you to stay fit and healthy, and deal with your Parkinson's disease at the same time. Many of you may already be on a restricted eating plan, such as a low-sodium, low-cholesterol, or diabetic diet. Before you undertake any new eating plan, weight-loss program, or fitness routine, be sure to discuss it with your physician.

Good Food for Good Health

Most Americans should change the way they eat. Our poor dietary habits contribute to the fact that we have among the highest rates of heart disease, stroke, and cancer in the industrialized world—and having Parkinson's disease does not make you immune to any of these conditions, especially as you get older. However, a "good-health consciousness" has swept the country in recent years. Even fast-food restaurants now offer low-fat alternatives to cholesterol-laden meals. If you haven't already jumped on the healthy-eating bandwagon, the time to come aboard is now.

Staying active and feeling well with Parkinson's disease require you to pay special attention to what you eat, how much, and at what times of the day. In the early stages of Parkinson's disease, many patients experience weight gain, resulting primarily from a decrease in activity but also due to depression or other emotional crises. During later stages of the disease, many patients lose weight as muscular rigidity affects their ability to chew and swallow properly. In addition, tremors and dyskinesias may burn off more energy than you take in with your diet. Later in this section you'll find out how to avoid such weight gain and loss.

The Principles of Protein Redistribution

It's important to understand the relationship between when you eat and when you take your medication. Since it is best to take Sinemet on an empty stomach, most people take their dose with a whole glass of water or juice about a half an hour before they eat their meals. If there is food in your stomach when you take Sinemet, it will take longer for the levodopa to be absorbed into the bloodstream and, therefore, longer for the medication to "kick in." When you first start taking Sinemet, however, you may feel a bit nauseated. Feel free to eat a few crackers when you take your pill if you need to settle your stomach.

As the disease progresses, the amount of protein you eat, and when you eat it, may become an issue. Levodopa is a naturally occurring substance called a large neutral amino acid, or LNAA. There are several different kinds of LNAAs in the protein foods we eat and digest, and the bloodstream transports them to different parts of the body. Levodopa, for instance, works to reduce PD symptoms only after it has been transported by the blood to the brain.

The bloodstream, however, can transport only a certain number of LNAAs—and only a limited number of these amino acids can cross the blood-brain barrier. The more protein you eat, the more LNAAs of all kinds will be in your bloodstream. Not only will it take longer for the levodopa to reach your brain, but more of it will be metabolized by the intestine or in the blood, producing no anti-Parkinson effects at all.

Many physicians feel that the wearing-off or the on-off effects of PD therapy may be caused, or at least exacerbated, by excess protein in the diet. If you experience these effects, you may want to consider reducing or at least redistributing your protein intake by avoiding protein-rich foods during the day, saving them instead for the evening meal. That way, Sinemet will be absorbed most efficiently when it is most needed.

Does this mean you must say good-bye forever to bacon and eggs? Perhaps in the morning. If protein intake is interfering with your levodopa absorption, you may well have to bid adieu to protein-rich breakfasts. Instead, substitute fresh fruit and low-protein cereals. But then feel free to have your former breakfast for dinner; that way, you'll be able to enjoy the food you love (admittedly at a new time) and still get the full benefits of your medication when you need them most. Remember, however, that the high fat content of your "breakfast for dinner" requires you to indulge in these foods only rarely.

The goal is not to eliminate all protein from your diet; indeed, a certain amount of protein is vital to proper body function; the United States Recommended Daily Allowance of protein ranges from between 30 to 50 grams. Table 3 will give you an idea of the protein content of some common foods.

Many people mistakenly think that protein exists mostly in meat, fish, and eggs, but you can see from Table 3 that most dairy

TABLE 3.
THE PROTEIN CONTENT OF COMMON FOODS

Item	Portion	Protein	Allowed on Diet
Almonds	⅔ cup	19 grams	no
Apples (juice)	1 medium	trace	yes
Asparagus	6–7 spears	2–3 grams	yes
Baby food (fruit)	3½ ounces	trace	yes
Baby food (vegs.)	3½ ounces	1–2 grams	yes
Bacon	2 strips	5 grams	no
Bananas	1 small	1 gram	yes
Beans—kidney	½ cup	6–8 grams	no
—lima	½ cup	6–8 grams	no
—snap green	½–¾ cup	1–2 grams	yes
—yellow	½–¾ cup	1–2 grams	yes
—wax	½–¾ cup	1–2 grams	yes
Beef	3½ ounces	14–27 grams	no
Beets	½ cup	1 gram	yes
Blueberries	⅔ cup	1 gram	yes
Bouillon	1 cube	trace	yes
Breads—wheat —white	1 slice	2 grams	yes
Breads—Italian —French	3½ ounces	9 grams	no
Breadcrumbs	sprinkle	trace	yes
Broccoli, cooked	⅔ cup	3 grams	yes
Butter	1 tablespoon	trace	yes
Buttermilk	½ cup	4 grams	yes
Cabbage	1⅔ cups	1 gram	yes
Cake	1 small piece	4 grams	no
Candy butterscotch caramels fudge hard candy marshmallows	1 ounce	0–1 gram	yes
Cantaloupe	5-inch diameter	1 gram	yes
Carrots	⅔ cup	1 gram	yes
Cauliflower	1 cup	2 grams	yes

TABLE 3. (*cont.*)
THE PROTEIN CONTENT OF COMMON FOODS

Item	Portion	Protein	Allowed on Diet
Celery	2 stalks	1 gram	yes
Chard	⅔ cup	2 grams	yes
Cheese	1 ounce	5–7 grams	no
blue			
cheddar			
Parmesan			
Swiss			
cottage			
Cream cheese	½ ounce	1 gram	yes
Cherries	½ cup	trace–1 gram	yes
sour			
red			
raw			
Maraschino			
Chicken	3½ ounces	22–32 grams	no
Chocolate	3½ ounces	11 grams	no
Chocolate syrup	1 tablespoon	trace	yes
Coleslaw	¾ cup	1 gram	yes
Cookies	1 cookie	1 gram	yes
Corn on the cob	1 small ear	3 grams	yes
Corn, cream-style	½ cup	2 grams	yes
Crabs	3½ ounces	17 grams	no
Crackers	2 crackers	1 gram	yes
graham			
saltine			
soda			
Cranberries	½ cup	trace	yes
Cucumbers	⅓ cuke	1 gram	yes
Custard	½ cup	5 grams	no
Dates, pitted	¼ cup	1 gram	yes
Doughnuts	1	5 grams	no
Eggplant	3½ ounces	1 gram	yes
Eggs, raw or cooked	1 medium	7 grams	no
Fats (oil)	½ cup	0 gram	yes
Figs	3 small	1 gram	yes
Fish	3½ ounces	20–82 grams	no

TABLE 3. (*cont.*)
THE PROTEIN CONTENT OF COMMON FOODS

Item	Portion	Protein	Allowed on Diet
Fruit cocktail	½ cup	trace	yes
Gelatin, dry	⅔ cup	86 grams	no
Grapefruit	½ small, juice	1 gram	yes
Grapes	1 bunch, ⅔ cup	1 gram	yes
Honey	1 tablespoon	trace	yes
Honeydew melon	1½-inch by 7-inch wedge	1 gram	yes
Ice cream, plain 12% fat	¾ cup	4 grams	no
Ice milk	⅔ cup	5 grams	no
Jams, jelly	1 tablespoon	trace	yes
Kidneys	3½ ounces	15–17 grams	no
Lamb	3 ounces	22 grams	no
Lemons, limes	1 whole	1 gram	yes
Lentils	3½ ounces	8 grams	no
Lettuce	4 large leaves	1 gram	yes
Liver, all types	3½ ounces	30 grams	no
Luncheon meats	3½ ounces	15 grams	no
Macaroni, pasta	⅔ cup	5 grams	yes
Milk	1 cup	8 grams	no
Olives	10–16	trace–1 gram	yes
Oranges	1 small	1 gram	yes
Pancakes	one 4-inch cake	2 grams	no
Potato pancake	1 pancake	trace–1 gram	yes
Peaches	½ cup, 1 small	trace	yes
Peanuts—roasted salted legumes	⅔ cup	26 grams	no
Peas	⅔ cup	5 grams	no
Peppers	1 large	1 gram	yes
Pickles	½ cup, 1 large	1 gram	yes
Pies	⅙ pie	6–11 grams	no
Pizza	⅙ of 14-inch pie	12 grams	no
Pineapple	1 medium slice or ¾ cup	trace	yes
Pine nuts	3½ ounces	13–31 grams	no

TABLE 3. (*cont.*)
The Protein Content of Common Foods

Item	Portion	Protein	Allowed on Diet
Popcorn	1 cup popped	2 grams	yes
Pork	3 ounces	22 grams	no
Potatoes	½ cup, 1 med.	2 grams	yes
Potato chips	10 medium or 7 large	1 gram	yes
Pretzels	5 small sticks	trace	yes
Prunes	⅔ cup	1–2 grams	yes
Radishes	4 small	trace	yes
Raisins	1 tablespoon only	trace	yes
Rice	⅓ cup only	1 gram	yes
Puffed rice cereal	1 cup	1 gram	yes
Salad dressing	3 tablespoons	trace–1 gram	yes
Sherbet	½ cup	1 gram	yes
Soup chicken noodle tomato (with water)	½ cup	1 gram	yes
Soybean products		9–47 grams	no
Spinach	½ cup	3 grams	no
Squash	½ cup	1 gram	yes
Strawberries	⅔ cup	1 gram	yes
Sugar		0 gram	yes
Tomatoes	1 small	1 gram	yes
Ketchup		trace	yes
Turkey	3½ ounces	30 grams	no
Turnip	⅔ cup	1 gram	yes
Veal	3½ ounces	26 grams	no
Vinegar	½ cup	0 gram	yes
Waffles	2 small	9 grams	no
Walnuts	½ cup	7 grams	no
Watermelon	3½ ounces	1 gram	yes
Yogurt	1 cup	8 grams	no

products, including milk, cheese, ice cream, and yogurt, also are rich in protein. So, too, are many cereals, flours, and even some vegetables. Generally speaking, any food listed with 2 grams or less of protein per serving can be consumed during the day on a protein-restricted diet, as long as the total amount of protein does not exceed 10 grams before 5:00 P.M.

If you feel that you would benefit from a protein redistribution plan, discuss the matter with your physician. Most PD patients, however, find that eating three well-balanced meals a day—one-half hour *after* taking their medication—does not interfere with the benefits of Sinemet or other anti-Parkinson drugs.

Vitamin Therapy

Many patients ask about vitamin supplements. Vitamins are substances required by the body in very small amounts. If you eat a balanced diet, you should be getting all the vitamins you need. If you are unable to eat enough, then taking a supplement may be warranted and will most likely do you no harm; contrary to popular belief, however, vitamins will not give you extra energy or increase your stamina in any way.

There is some controversial evidence, however, that vitamin C and vitamin E may help reduce the PD symptoms and even retard the progression of the disease. As you may recall, substances called free radicals are produced by the various metabolic processes that take place in the brain. These free radicals are capable of causing damage to nerve cells, including those in the substantia nigra. Levodopa therapy for Parkinson's disease itself may also cause an increase in the production of free radicals, leading a few researchers to believe that some anti-Parkinson drugs themselves may hasten the progression of the disease. This is a very controversial point. Certain other substances, called antioxidants, are known to break down free radicals or prevent their formation. Vitamin E and vitamin C are known to be antioxidants; studies are now under way to find out if they will indeed prove to be effective in the treatment of PD by slowing the progression of the disease. Before you take more than the recommended daily dosages of these vitamins, please discuss the matter with your physician.

The Principles of Good Nutrition

How many of us—healthy or ill—know what a well-balanced meal really consists of? Learning a bit about proper nutrition and following a sound eating plan will keep your body in better condition, thereby helping you better cope with the effects and side effects of PD.

According to the American Heart Association, a typical modern American now obtains more than 40 percent of his calories from fat, about 20 percent from complex carbohydrates (vegetables, grains, and fibers), 20 percent from sugar, and the other 20 percent from protein. Changing the above percentages may go a long way toward helping you to maintain proper body weight and a healthy heart and circulatory system. The American Heart Association recommends the following:

1. Total fat intake should be less than 30 percent of calories; of this percentage, only 10 percent should consist of saturated fats (whole milk, some cheeses, butter, meats, cream, hydrogenated vegetable shortening).
2. Cholesterol intake should be less than 100 mg per 1,000 calories; not to exceed 300 mg per day.
3. Protein intake should add up to no more than 15 percent of each day's calories.
4. Carbohydrate intake should constitute 50 to 55 percent or more of calories, with emphasis on increasing complex carbohydrates such as grains and legumes.
5. Sodium intake should be reduced to approximately 3 grams a day.
6. Alcohol intake should be limited to 15 percent of total calories and not exceed 50 ml of ethanol per day (about 2 ounces of liquor or 2 glasses of beer).
7. Total calories should be sufficient to maintain proper body weight.
8. A wide variety of foods should be consumed.

The old adage "everything in moderation" turns out to be remarkably accurate—and it holds true for Parkinson's disease patients as well. A glass of wine or a cocktail should pose no problem for most patients, nor should an occasional piece of cake or other dessert.

It is important to keep in mind that the symptoms and side effects of PD may very well have an impact on the way you eat and the way you metabolize your food. Indeed, maintaining proper body weight may become a challenge for you, but one you should try your best to meet. Table 4, prepared by Metropolitan Life Insurance, gives you a rough idea of what you should weigh depending on your height.

Where do you fit in? If you find your weight is much above or below these guidelines, check with your physician to see if he or she thinks you need a special diet.

Avoiding Weight Loss

The psychological and physical aspects of Parkinson's disease may reduce a patient's ability to eat enough of the right kinds of food. Several factors contribute to this. For one thing, many patients simply no longer enjoy eating. There is some evidence that the imbalance of neurotransmitters in the PD brain may contribute to a decrease in appetite. The fact that many patients are no longer physically active may be another factor. In addition, the stress and fear felt by many patients with a chronic illness may not only lessen appetite but also put increased demands on the body. Other psychological factors, including depression, may also reduce the desire to eat.

In many cases of advanced disease, tremors, bradykinesia, and an impaired ability to swallow make eating both difficult and unappealing. Severe tremors and dyskinesias can actually burn extra calories; in fact, some patients may have to increase the amount of calories they consume during the day to compensate. In Chapter Seven, you'll learn some tips on how to chew, swallow, and use utensils should PD symptoms begin to prevent you from obtaining proper nutrition.

In the meantime, if you're having difficulty chewing and swallowing, remember to take your time when eating. Feeling rushed will only increase your symptoms and lessen your enjoyment of the food itself. Some patients have found that using a heating tray to keep foods warm longer will take some of the pressure off.

TABLE 4.
DESIRABLE WEIGHT FOR HEIGHT

MEN

Height	Small Frame	Medium Frame	Large Frame
5'2"	112–120	118–129	126–141
5'3"	115–123	121–133	129–144
5'4"	118–126	124–136	132–148
5'5"	121–129	127–139	135–152
5'6"	124–133	130–143	138–156
5'7"	128–137	134–147	142–161
5'8"	132–141	138–152	147–166
5'9"	136–145	142–156	151–170
5'10"	140–150	146–160	155–174
5'11"	144–154	150–165	159–179
6'	148–158	154–170	164–184
6'1"	152–162	158–175	168–189
6'2"	156–167	162–180	173–194
6'3"	160–171	167–185	178–199
6'4"	164–175	172–190	182–204

WOMEN

Height	Small Frame	Medium Frame	Large Frame
4'10"	92–98	96–101	104–119
4'11"	94–101	98–110	106–122
5'	96–104	101–113	109–125
5'1"	99–107	104–116	112–128
5'2"	102–110	107–119	115–131
5'3"	105–113	110–122	118–134
5'4"	108–116	113–126	121–138
5'5"	111–119	116–130	125–142
5'6"	114–123	120–135	129–146
5'7"	118–127	124–139	133–150
5'8"	122–131	128–143	137–154
5'9"	126–135	132–147	141–158
5'10"	130–140	136–151	145–163
5'11"	134–144	140–155	149–168
6'	138–148	144–159	153–173

Source: Metropolitan Life.

Instead of eating three large meals a day, some patients find that smaller snacks taken several times during the day are more appealing.

If you begin losing weight, see your doctor. He or she may evaluate you for other causes of weight loss, prescribe food supplements, or suggest drinking milk shakes, eggnogs, and other calorie-rich foods to bolster your caloric intake. Adding sour cream, butter, and other condiments—if fat and cholesterol are not problems for you—may also help bolster your diet.

Please remember: It is important for you to get enough vitamins, minerals, and other nutrients. With malnutrition comes a susceptibility to infection, delayed recovery time from minor illnesses, increased muscular weakness, and a tendency to develop pressure sores if you are wheelchair-bound or bedridden.

Avoiding Weight Gain

Hunger is only one of many reasons we consume food: boredom, frustration, stress, depression, and excitement are just a few of the nonhunger-related reasons for eating.

"The fact that I have a lifelong chronic illness often seems a perfectly justifiable reason to consume three pieces of chocolate cake while I watch soap operas in the afternoon," laughs Margaret, the retired schoolteacher whose case history you read in the last chapter. "But when I gained five pounds in the first few months after I was diagnosed, I knew I had to watch it."

For those of you who have gained weight recently or who were overweight before you were diagnosed with PD, now is the time to get yourself back in shape. The key to successful weight loss is finding a flexible, easy-to-follow eating plan that offers a wide variety of foods. To lose weight sensibly, consume no more than about 1,200 to 1,800 calories per day; if you keep your intake at this level you should be able to lose about one to two pounds a week, safely and steadily.

For most people, however, the task of counting calories and calculating what percentage of these calories consist of proteins, carbohydrates, or fats is troublesome and complicated. A simpler method is to go back to the old-fashioned "four basic food groups" idea. Both the American Heart Association and reputable diet programs such as Weight Watchers recommend the following daily portions of fruits, vegetables, breads, protein, dairy products, and fat as a sensible eating plan for weight loss:

- 4–6 ounces protein (chicken, turkey, fish, lean beef, veal, pork, lamb, lentils, dried peas, nuts; this includes egg whites as desired; but only 3-4 whole eggs per week)
- 3 servings of one-half cup (or more) of fresh vegetables
- 3 servings of medium-sized fruit
- 4 servings of bread/starches, about 80 to 100 calories per serving (bread, English muffins, pasta, cereal, potatoes, rice, popcorn, starchy vegetables such as acorn squash, corn, peas)
- 2 8-ounce servings of low-fat milk, yogurt, or cottage cheese (this includes hard cheese, but no more than 4 1-ounce servings per week)
- no more than 2 tablespoons of fat (butter, olive or vegetable oil)

By using this plan, you'll replace the often tedious struggle with calories and "dieting" with the more natural approach of portion control and food variety. Another key ingredient is water: consume at least 8 glasses of water a day. It not only will bolster your weight loss efforts but will also help you absorb medication better and help control side effects such as constipation and dry mouth.

Keep in mind that there is virtually no food forever denied to you: a piece of cake or a thick juicy steak can be an *occasional* indulgence, even for those watching their weight or protein intake. By all means, enjoy the sensuous pleasure of eating delicious and nutritious food. Your life as a Parkinson's disease patient may be restricted in certain ways, but as long as you remain within sensible caloric and nutritional limits, feel free to enjoy your food to the fullest.

The Joy of Fitness

Maintaining proper body weight. Staying strong. Finding a balance between high stress and total exhaustion. What is the one thing that addresses all three health goals? Exercise—walking, jogging, stretching, swimming, whatever will get your heart pumping and your body moving.

If you have Parkinson's disease, it's more important than ever that you get your muscles moving, and keep them moving every day. Although bradykinesia, rigidity, and tremor may seem ample excuses not to exercise, the stiffness and slowness you feel from the disease process may only get worse more quickly if you don't lengthen and stretch your muscles.

In addition to alleviating some of your PD symptoms, regular exercise will improve your overall physical and mental health. Exercise will help your heart and lungs work more efficiently, reducing the risk of heart problems. Your weight and cholesterol level are more easily controlled if physical activity is a part of your daily life. The more you exercise, the better you'll sleep, handle stress, and fight off disease.

Equally important to someone suffering from a chronic illness are the psychological benefits of exercise. If you stick to a routine and meet new challenges, your self-esteem is sure to increase. Low-level depression, so often an unwanted side effect of chronic illness, is relieved by physical activity; in fact, the process of exercise releases chemicals called endorphins, which give you a kind of psychological high, helping you to feel less tired and more energetic. Joining a gym, taking sailing lessons, or playing a sport also alleviates some of the social isolation experienced by many PD patients who tend to withdraw even from their friends and family.

Again, every PD patient will be affected by the process of Parkinson's disease in a different way. Some patients mountain climb, deep-sea fish, and take aerobics classes for years after diagnosis. Others are restricted early in their disease process and must replace more strenuous activities with ones that require less agility and coordination.

Except those with advanced disease and/or with severe balance problems, almost everyone can enjoy some sort of workout. For those of you who have been athletic in the past, Parkinson's disease may eventually limit your activities. However, most patients find that they can still pursue their favorite activities if special accommodations are made.

"I'm no longer the runner-up in the Over 50 Singles Championships," Maureen, a 59-year-old PD patient, admits. "But if I'm careful, I can still play a set or two of tennis with an understanding competitor. If I'm feeling off, if I'm nervous that I'll fall if I try to pivot, I won't play a game. Instead, I'll spend a half hour or so hitting the ball against the backboard."

Jackson, 73 years old and a PD patient for six years, boasts that he hasn't missed a Wednesday golf game for twelve years. "I was never very good—and now I'm a little worse—but I love the game. Most of the time I walk the course, at least the first nine holes. That way I get in some real exercise at the same time that I'm smacking the ball."

If you, like Maureen or Jackson, are already an experienced athlete in one sport or another, by all means, keep it up. The part of the motor control system damaged by PD makes automatic movements—walking, getting out of a chair, crossing one's legs— more difficult. Learned or acquired skills, on the other hand, are apt to be less affected by parkinsonism.

If you've never been physically active, you might find it difficult to start and keep to a regular daily exercise regimen. Of course, the more you enjoy an activity, the more likely you'll make it a part of your life. Some people find exercising with a partner more fun; it provides support, encouragement, and company.

"When my wife's doctor told her she needed to exercise every day," recalls Larry, the 56-year-old husband of a PD patient, "we went out and bought an indoor exercise bike. She used it regularly for about a week, then it kind of ended up in the closet, like it does for most people, I guess. Our solution is to take a long walk every night after dinner, just the two of us. She's pretty slow and stiff these days, and sometimes pretty shaky, but we try to do a mile in about 40 to 45 minutes on our good nights, an hour on our bad. Not only does Laura feel better, but so do I. I've lost a little of my none-too-attractive spare tire and really look forward to that quiet time with just my wife and the fresh air."

One way to increase your daily activity level is to substitute the active for the passive: climbing stairs instead of taking an elevator, walking to the store for the newspaper rather than having it delivered, washing the dishes by hand rather than by machine, etc. You'd be surprised how much simple daily chores such as vacuuming and dusting, done conscientiously and with vigor, exercise your body. For most people, even those who've never been athletic, the more they stretch and strengthen their muscles, the better they feel. And the better they feel, the more they want to exercise.

Almost all general exercise programs, including those designed for the PD patient, center on three basic goals: attaining or maintaining cardiovascular health, muscle flexibility, and muscle strength. As long as you are able, you should try to achieve all three every day. A patient who only walks, for instance, even for several miles a day, may still have difficulty getting out of bed if he or she doesn't stretch and strengthen the other muscles of the body. Those who lift weights but never stretch may be only making matters worse, since their muscles are often tight enough due to the disease process.

Sticking to a Fitness Routine

- First, consult your physician before you begin. Make sure that what you are planning is both safe and beneficial.
- Set reasonable goals for yourself. Even if you've been active before, PD will no doubt affect your stamina and mobility. A physical therapist can be very helpful in assessing your capabilities and in planning a routine that will help you progress. Start slowly and build up gradually. Most important, don't expect to see results overnight.
- Schedule your daily exercise as if it were a doctor's appointment or other equally important commitment. Choose the time of day when you feel most "on," when you are experiencing the full benefits of your medication. PD patients should spend at least 15 minutes *every day* stretching and strengthening their muscles (see the PD Daily Dozen below). Cardiovascular activities should be performed three times a week for 30 minutes or more at each session.
- Structure your program to include adequate rest periods, or divide your program into several shorter sessions.
- Make sure you have proper equipment, including the right kind of shoes and clothing. Some patients, especially those with freezing or other gait disturbances, find that sneakers or other rubber-soled shoes stick to the floor or sidewalk, making it more difficult to walk or move. Instead, try a low-heeled

leather-soled walking shoe, even for playing sports. Check with a physical therapist for more advice.

- Before doing any kind of exercise, make sure you spend at least five to ten minutes warming up and doing gentle stretching. A good warm-up will prepare your heart and lungs for the upcoming activity, loosen your muscles and joints, and get the blood flowing to your muscles, all of which will help reduce the risk of injury due to pulls and sprains.
- If you experience any dizziness or pain, or if you have any trouble breathing, stop exercising immediately. If symptoms persist for more than a few minutes, contact your physician.

Working the Heart

Most exercise routines geared to the PD patient focus on maintaining range of mobility and muscle strength, since these factors are the ones most affected by the progress of the disease. Later in this chapter, you'll learn a series of daily exercises to increase muscular flexibility. It is important, however, that you don't neglect the health of your heart and circulatory system, especially as you age.

How does aerobic exercise improve your health? One link is between exercise and weight maintenance—the more you exercise, the more calories you burn. In addition, a number of studies have found that regular, vigorous exercise can lower total blood cholesterol, thereby reducing the risk for atherosclerosis, heart attack, and stroke. Diabetics who exercise regularly are often able to reduce their medication dramatically.

Your heart also benefits from a good workout. Because your muscles need more oxygen when they're at work, the heart must pump harder to get extra oxygen-rich blood to them. Normally, the heart pumps about 6 quarts of blood per minute in an average adult man, but when the body is exercising, blood volume to and from the heart rises to about 25 quarts per minute. This extra work strengthens the heart; the stronger it is, the less hard it has to work to meet the body's need for oxygen. Exercise also helps improve the health of the entire circulatory system because blood is distributed more evenly to all the blood vessels.

Before you start an aerobic exercise program, check with your physician and/or a physical therapist who specializes in working with PD patients. They will be able to tell if the disease has affected your balance or muscular strength to the degree that jogging or bicycling would be dangerous to you. Your doctor also may recommend a stress test to see how well your heart and blood vessels are functioning. A stress test involves having your heart rate measured by an electrocardiogram (ECG) and your blood pressure monitored by a technician while you jog on a treadmill or ride a stationary bicycle. A stress test will help diagnose heart disease through changes in the ECG. It will also help determine the amount of exercise your heart and muscles can handle without any adverse affects.

Based on the results of your stress test, your physician will give you your "target heart rate," or the rate at which your heart must work to provide health benefits to the cardiovascular system. Generally speaking, your target heart rate is between 70 and 85 percent of your maximum heart rate (your maximum heart rate is calculated by subtracting your age from 220). If you are 65 years old, then, your maximum heart rate would be 220 minus 60, or 160. Your target heart rate is between 112 and 136 beats per minute.

You can determine whether you are within your target zone by taking your pulse immediately after exercise. Place two fingers (*not* your thumb—it is also a pulse point and can disturb the accuracy of your reading) on one of your carotid arteries, located on the left or right of your throat in the neck. Count the beats for ten seconds, then multiply that number by 6. If your pulse rate is below the target range, you should increase either the intensity or the duration of your workout. If your pulse is above your target rate, slow down.

How often should you exercise? The optimal frequency for those beginning an exercise program is three or four times per week. Each period of exercise should last from 30 to 40 minutes each, which includes a 5- to 10-minute warm-up and 5- to 10-minute cool-down. Beginners should start out exercising for just 5 to 10 minutes, slowly increasing the amount of time until the target rate is reached.

What kinds of aerobic exercise can a patient with PD safely perform? Like so many other aspects of this disease, it all depends on the patient. As long as your balance is not affected, choose any aerobic exercise you enjoy performing. If you've been an avid jogger and still have no significant balance or freezing problems, there is no reason you can't continue your routine. Some patients find swimming to be therapeutic—it gives your cardiovascular system a workout while passively stretching nearly all the muscles of your body. (Please note: *Never* swim alone. PD patients with bradykinesia may find themselves "frozen" in the water, unable to swim to the edge of the pool or to shore, and will need help from a partner or lifeguard. In addition, balance problems can upset even those wading in shallow water; falls are equally dangerous in the water.)

Bicycling, either indoors or out, is also a good form of aerobic exercise. A new product on the market is the recumbent stationary bike; it allows you to lean against a seat back and use just your legs to pedal. This alleviates any pressure on the lower back and requires very little balance—a boon for the PD patient. Again, it is always best to exercise with a partner in case you need help in any way, especially if you have difficulty getting on or off exercise equipment.

A Word About Walking

Walking is one of the simplest, most inexpensive and pleasurable forms of exercise. Even if bradykinesia and rigidity have got the best of you, walking slowly, with the help of a willing companion, will lengthen and strengthen your leg muscles. If you're able to swing your arms, the muscles of your upper body get a good workout as well. Walking at a steady rate for a half an hour or more will raise your heart rate as well, giving your cardiovascular system a much needed boost.

If you have trouble walking due to balance problems, shuffling, and/or freezing, try the following hints:

1. Choose the right footwear—and most of you should leave "designer" sneakers and running shoes behind. Instead, choose a good walking shoe with firm arch support and a small heel. This will help keep you from slipping on the pavement.

2. When walking or standing, your feet should be spread apart approximately 10 inches. This will help you maintain better balance. Do not allow your feet to cross.
3. Exaggerate lifting your feet, as if you are marching. This avoids the tendency of many PD patients to shuffle and scuff. To help improve the height of your gait, practice stepping over a low object such as a phone book placed on the floor. Remember to concentrate on lifting toes when walking to avoid tripping.
4. Consciously exaggerate your normal arm swing when walking. This improves the cadence of walking and helps you both look and feel less rigid. To help strengthen your arm muscles, you can hold a rolled magazine in each hand or use wrist or hand weights.
5. Take as long steps as possible when walking. This can be accentuated by placing magazines or other objects on the floor and trying to walk over them without stepping on them.
6. Music makes any exercise easier to bear. It is often helpful to walk or march to music in an effort to establish an even, brisk walking rhythm.
7. When turning, never pivot in one spot. Instead, think of making a U-turn. Keep your feet apart and make the turn in a large arc and always in a forward direction. Again, remember to keep your feet from crossing in front of you.
8. Every once in a while, check your posture in a mirror. If you are tilted to the side or bent over, try to correct your posture as much as possible. Some people lean back against a wall until every part of the body, from the back of their heels and calves to the back of their head, is pressing against the surface. Then, make an effort to maintain a tall, erect posture while walking.
9. If you start taking rapid steps either forward or backward, stop yourself before you lose your balance. Once you've righted yourself, start walking again with high, long steps.

More tips on walking and on controlling other gait disturbances such as festination and retropulsion are covered in more depth in the A to Z Guide in Chapter Seven. Walking is indeed one of the best and most pleasurable ways to exercise your muscles, work your cardiovascular system, and perhaps most important of all, relax all the tension you hold in your head and heart.

Muscle Flexibility and Strength: Principles of Physical Therapy

No matter your age or the stage of your disease, once you've been diagnosed with Parkinson's disease, it is a good idea to see a professional physical therapist (PT). Physical therapy is a health profession that focuses on identifying, assessing, and correcting movement dysfunction.

As you know, the most problematic symptoms of PD are those related to movement: loss of flexibility, difficulty in walking and changing position, poor posture, stiffness. The first step is for the PT to perform a thorough examination of your muscle strength, length, and flexibility, much the same way as your physician did when he first rated the level of your disease. In addition, the PT will want to know how your condition affects your day-to-day functioning: Can you turn over and get out of bed? Sit and stand upright, with good posture? (You'll learn some PT tips to manage these and other activities in the A to Z Guide.)

Based on the results of his or her examination, the PT will then develop an exercise program that addresses your particular needs, strengths, and weaknesses. Most important, however, a PT will help you make sure that every one of your muscles is put through its full range of motion during your workout. Parkinson's disease can affect nearly every muscle in your body, from those controlling your smile to those that allow you to wiggle your toes.

Some patients see a PT, at home or at the hospital, once a week or once a month. Others visit less regularly for an occasional reevaluation or for advice on new problems or symptoms. If you think you would benefit from seeing a professional physical therapist, ask your physician to recommend one.

In the meantime, you should perform the following exercises every day. Chosen because they stretch the major muscle groups most affected by Parkinson's disease, they'll give you a relatively quick, head-to-toe workout. Please note, however, that they represent the *minimum* amount of physical activity you should attain; feel free to supplement them with other exercise routines devised by a physical therapist or described in literature from the American Parkinson's Disease Association.

For those of you with a videocassette recorder, a number of videotapes, including "Rhythms and Moves: Therapeutic Home Exercise Program for Parkinsonians," devised by Paula Benoist Falwell, PT, specialize in stretching and flexibility exercises for the PD patient. (Please see Appendix I for more information.)

The PD Daily Dozen

REPEAT ALL EXERCISES TEN TIMES.

Chin Tuck
1. Sit up straight, with shoulders back and relaxed, and eyes straight ahead (start position). Notice position of your head: it probably is slightly forward, with your earlobe well in front of the middle of your shoulder.
2. Tuck your chin under and glide head backward and try to align your earlobe with the middle of your shoulders. Hold for 5 seconds.

Head Tilts
1. Start position as for chin tuck.
2. Tilt head down toward your right shoulder; keep your nose and eyes straight head.
3. Place your right hand on the side of your head and *gently* pull your head closer to your shoulder, thereby stretching your neck muscles further. Stretch only as much as is comfortable for you; you should feel no pain.
4. With your right hand, push your left shoulder down toward the floor, further stretching your neck muscles.
   Repeat this exercise on the left side.

Head Turns
1. Start position as for chin tuck.
2. Turn your head to the right.
3. Nod head down toward your shoulder three times.
   Repeat exercise on the left side.

Trunk Bends, Forward and Back

1. While seated, place feet on the outside of a chair, hold on to front seat edge with both hands. Bend trunk forward toward your knees keeping your bottom down on the seat.
2. Straighten up, place hands behind your head, and lean trunk back over the back of the chair.

Trunk Bends, Side to Side

1. While seated, place hands on back legs of a chair. Bend to the right side, sliding your right hand down along the back leg, while your left arm comes up along the back of the chair.
   Repeat to opposite side.

Trunk Twists

1. While seated, place your feet on the outside of your chair. Place both hands on the back of the chair. Gently twist to the right side.
   Repeat to the left.

Hip Stretch

1. Start position: While seated, place right ankle on left thigh.
2. Push right knee down toward the floor; try to make your shin parallel to the floor.
3. Clasp hands around your right knee and pull knee up toward your chest and left shoulder.
   Repeat on left side.

Hamstring Stretch

1. Start position: Sit back in one chair with your legs straight across and resting on another chair. Your feet should be together, toes up, and your knees slightly bent.
2. Push your knees down (toward the floor) and flex your feet. Hold for 5 seconds.
3. Add thigh strengthening by then raising first your left and then your right leg straight up off the chair.

Shoulder Stretch

1. Start position: While seated, clasp hands behind your back.

2. Roll shoulders back, straighten elbows, and push arms back as far as possible; hold for 3 seconds.

Shoulder Raises
1. Start position: While seated, clasp hands behind your back.
2. Raise hands up along the back of the chair.

Facial Mobility
1. Say "eee."
2. Hold that smile for the rest of the day.

Arm Stretch
1. Stretch your arms out to the side at shoulder level.
2. Cross arms around your chest and give yourself a big hug. You deserve it for all your hard work.
3. Share your exercises with your friends and family and hug somebody you love.

Chapter Six

Coming to Terms with Chronic Illness

Just as everyone will experience the physical symptoms of Parkinson's disease differently, so too will they learn to accept and cope with their illness at different rates and in uniquely individual ways. In this chapter, the range of emotions and coping skills common to those suffering from chronic illness is outlined. No doubt your unique spirit will pave its own path through the course of your disease, but you may find parallels to your own experience and gain insight into the road ahead.

It's important that you know you're not alone in your fears and your hopes. If you've just learned that you have Parkinson's disease, or if your condition has recently worsened, for instance, you may be feeling afraid and helpless, just as Margaret, the retired schoolteacher, did when she first heard that she had PD.

"At first, I couldn't stand it. I shut myself away completely. My husband had died a year before and I was just learning to be on my own," Margaret recalls. "When the doctor told me I had Parkinson's disease, I felt alone, helpless, and ugly. It felt like I was dying. I didn't tell another soul for almost two months."

Any chronic illness, but especially one that limits your mobility and affects your appearance the way PD often does, may bring with it a profound loss of self-esteem. The physical changes that result from the disease or medication side effects include a loss of muscle tone and fat, dermatological changes such as dry, flaky skin, and a stooped posture and shuffling walk: all conditions commonly associated with old age. Most Parkinson's patients, however, receive their diagnosis in their early 60s, sometimes earlier, long before these changes might otherwise have occurred. It often leaves them feeling unattractive and "old before their time."

"My first thought when I heard the diagnosis was 'PD is an old people's disease. And I'm not old,' " Ellen, a 52-year-old woman diagnosed a year ago, remembers. "But then I thought about how stiff I felt, how slow I was getting around, how bent my posture had become. And I *felt* old, and alone. I didn't want to be around 'healthy' people because I felt like damaged goods or something."

This lack of self-esteem and self-confidence stems not only from the physical and cosmetic aspects of Parkinson's disease, but also from an anticipated loss of independence. It doesn't matter if you've been a breadwinner or a homemaker, your confidence in your ability to perform your daily activities is likely to be diminished—even if your disease is very mild.

"Suddenly, I had limits. I guess that's what hit me first," recalls Alan, the advertising executive you first met in Chapter One. "I was just 54 and it felt like my whole life was over. With the diagnosis, I thought, 'I'll never be able to work again, I won't be able to ski next winter,' etc. Now, two years later, I realize that many of those fears were unfounded, but I'll never forget how real they were at the time."

Another injury to self-esteem comes from realizing that you may soon have to depend on other people, at least for some of your needs. Although many PD patients live on their own or with minimal support for some years after diagnosis, fear of dependence is an overriding concern for most patients. This is especially true when the diagnosis is first made and ignorance about its variable course is common.

"When I realized I would probably have to move in with my daughter, I was devastated. I always swore I'd never be a burden on my child," Margaret admits. "Well, it ended up not being so awful. First of all, I lived on my own for almost two years after my diagnosis. And second, I still care for myself most of the time and actually have been a help to my daughter and her family. We have a wonderful new give-and-take relationship and, in some ways, my disease has made this possible. I know it will become more difficult for everyone as my PD progresses, but we just take one day at a time for now."

Related to the fear of dependency are financial and employment considerations. Many patients are still actively employed when they receive their diagnosis and worry about their ability to keep their jobs until they are able to retire. Income-producing skills may be hampered, and disability payments, savings funds, and pensions may be limited.

"All I can think of is my family and the house. I still have two kids in college and a wife to support," admits Larry, a 60-year-old lawyer with his own practice. "I wonder about being able to keep up my private insurance payments. Even now, my medicine is putting a strain on our budget. I just have to keep working. That's the most important thing."

A Maze of Emotions

Like most other newly diagnosed patients, Larry has about a million different thoughts and worries swirling through his head. The variety of emotions accompanying the diagnosis of Parkinson's disease is vast, complex, and persistent; you may think you've put aside your anger or depression once and for all, only to have it spring back at you months or years later. At one time or another, most patients report feeling overwhelmed by their emotions.

Although many things about Parkinson's disease are unpredictable, how you as an individual will cope with your condition may not be one of them. Generally speaking, you'll react to the many emotional and physical demands of PD the same way you've handled crises and challenges in the past. Are you an optimistic, ambitious person? If so, chances are you'll attack your disease with equal hope and energy. If you're a pessimist, you'll know that your situation is *never* as bad as you think it will be and it probably won't be with PD either.

Most psychologists liken the emotional responses to a diagnosis of chronic illness to the reaction to a terminal disease or even a death. We don't respond all at once, but rather in various stages process the information and its effects on our lives. It is likely that you'll experience one or all of the following emotions at some point during the course of the disease:

Shock: Mercifully, nature provides you with a blanket of numbness to protect you from bad news. In other words, your first reaction may be no reaction at all. This period of shock allows you and your family a moment of "calm before the storm," so to speak.

Denial: After the initial shock, you may attempt to deny the diagnosis altogether, especially if the disease is still in its early stages. Many PD patients who experience tremor as a major symptom, for instance, will continue to insist that it's caused by stress or that it's all in their imagination. Some patients accept the diagnosis itself, but deny the prognosis: They think they can "beat" the disease and its progression.

"I was sure I could control it, that it would never get any worse," Hugh admits. "Especially because I'm so young, I thought I could exercise it away or take care of myself so well that my rigidity and tremor wouldn't progress. In a way, I still feel like that and, frankly, I think it's helped." Indeed, denial is not all negative: It offers both the patient and the family a way to escape the overwhelming aspects of the disability and learn about the long-range effects slowly.

Reaction: After the denial stage has initially passed, the emotions of a PD patient run the gamut from anxiety to fear and to depression. Many patients react with pure, undistilled anger. Unfortunately this anger is not always directed at the disease.

"I don't think she wants to remember this, but when my mother first fully realized she had PD, she started acting very hostile both to me and to her doctor," Mariella, Margaret's daughter, describes. "This normally sweet, very intelligent and kind woman would literally yell at the doctor over the telephone if he hadn't called in a prescription to the pharmacy on time or some other minor infraction. She nagged at me constantly, often in a very bitter way."

Like Margaret, many patients direct their frustration with the disease at the medical profession, irrationally (but quite normally) blaming the messenger for the bad news. In addition, the fact that Margaret also lashed out at Mariella is most likely related to her growing fears of dependency. This anxiety is often related, at least in part, to a lack of patient education at the onset of the disease. Many people remember an affected acquaintance or relative whose

PD struck before drug therapy was available and see only a future of helpless dependency for themselves as well.

Some patients may in fact feel so overwhelmed by their circumstances that they regress, making childlike demands on spouses and family members and reacting to new situations with emotional immaturity. The family, in an effort to comfort the patient, may assume responsibilities that the patient could maintain, if pushed to do so. Such a vicious cycle renders the patient far more dependent than need be.

Unfortunately, however, most patients will eventually be forced to give up some measure of independence as the disease progresses. There's no getting around the fact that your life has changed in some fundamental ways. If you're like most PD patients, you've started to think about retiring, hopefully with enough money and good health to travel or pursue projects you've put off during your working years. Younger patients have even more concerns about their future, perhaps having young children still to raise and careers to maintain. Although there is no reason to think that such plans must now be scrapped entirely, adjustments may have to be made.

When patients realize the potential effects of PD, they often feel a profound sense of loss: a loss of their former healthy selves and the lives they hoped to lead in the future. It is perfectly normal to grieve over that loss, and your family members and friends may grieve with you. You might find yourself crying often as you long for the self you consider to have been lost to Parkinson's disease.

Such feelings are related to one of the toughest and most recurring emotional problems experienced by the patient: depression. Faced with a loss of self-esteem and self-confidence, a loss of independence, grief over what might have been, as well as the physical realities of a degenerative disease, it is no wonder that many patients sink into periods of deep unhappiness and withdrawal. In addition, there is some evidence that the disease process itself may cause depression in some patients.

Although depression is a normal coping stage and may recur at any time during the course of the disease, when depression lasts for more than a few weeks or disrupts basic, day-to-day functioning, some form of therapeutic intervention may be necessary. (See the A to Z Guide for more details.)

Mobilization: There will come a time, perhaps even before you've passed through all the reaction stages, when you say to yourself and to your loved ones: "I want to live. . . . Show me how." Since you're reading this book, we'll assume that you've already reached this point. You're eager to learn how to better manage your disease, and it's important that you get your family and friends to join in as much as possible, too. Again, you may lose this feeling from time to time, only to become reinspired at a later stage.

"About eight months after my diagnosis," remembers Alan, "I started to read everything about Parkinson's disease I could get my hands on. I brought lists and lists of questions to ask my doctor. Then, I met a patient who had had PD for about fifteen years. He was quite severely disabled, in a wheelchair, tremoring uncontrollably, almost unable to speak. I totally shut down. I didn't want to learn any more about it. If that was my future, I just didn't want to know. I'm just now starting to put my feelers out for information again."

Accommodation: A lifelong process of change and acceptance, accommodation begins when both the patient and family understand, as much as possible, the disabling characteristics of PD and agree to work together to adapt to them. Thanks to drug therapy, most people are able to enjoy quite normal lives for many years—as long as they are willing to accommodate certain changes in their routines necessitated by their disease.

"I was your quintessential homemaker," Laura claims with a laugh. "I knitted sweaters for my kids and grandkids, sewed all my own clothes, even made lace doilies for my bridge club. But pretty soon my tremor and stiffness in my hands made it impossible to do much of anything. Then my daughter came up with a great compromise. She and I would shop together for the patterns and the fabric, then she would cut the fabric out and help me pin the hems. My right leg worked fine, so I could use a sewing machine without much trouble. It wasn't everything, but it was pretty good. I adapted."

As Laura's story illustrates, accommodation can rarely be accomplished alone. Neither, in fact, can any other aspects of coping with chronic illness. Whether you like it or not, you are not the only one who will experience Parkinson's disease: Everyone you know and love will be affected, too. As you deal with your emotions, never forget that the people around you—your spouse or life partner, your family and friends—will be experiencing similar feelings of anger, denial, grief, and acceptance. You must offer them support and information that will help them cope with the reality of your chronic illness and its effect on all your lives.

How Do I Tell Them?

"Hindsight may be the better part of valor," 48-year-old Chuck recalls, "but if I could do something differently, it would be to let more people in on my situation earlier on, maybe even before I got the actual diagnosis." A technical writer for a large chemical company, Chuck kept his condition a secret for as long as he could. "I think if I'd just said to my boss, 'I haven't been feeling well. I'm going to see a doctor,' then clued him in on the progress, it might have been easier on both of us. Instead, it all had to come out at once and maybe seemed more of a big deal than it needed to be, especially since I was still in shock a bit, too. Luckily, he was really supportive anyway, but it might have gone even smoother if he'd been in on it from the start, like my wife was. In fact, my boss was relieved that I had Parkinson's disease. He thought I had a drinking or drug problem."

Indeed, as hard as you deny—even to yourself—your early symptoms or try to hide your condition after you receive the diagnosis, other people are bound to have noticed something amiss. Most patients find that it is best to tell the people in their lives that they have PD as soon as possible. The more you try to protect the people you love from knowing about your physical symptoms or emotional side effects, the farther away from you will they grow.

Yes, relationships will change. Strong marriages may become even stronger; weak ones may break apart. Friendships built on solid foundations of respect and mutual interests will most likely flourish with the addition of a new challenge. Employers are often reassured, as Chuck's was, that a difficulty in balance or walking is the result of a treatable chronic illness, and not from the use of alcohol or drugs. However, although it is illegal to do so, some employers find ways of terminating employment. If there is any doubt about how an employer may react, it may be beneficial to check with a lawyer before you approach the situation.

Establishing a network of supportive friends and family is a key ingredient in the treatment of Parkinson's disease. You will probably experience a great sense of relief once the news is finally out in the open.

Telling the Children

Young children whose parents or other relatives have a chronic disease such as Parkinson's should be told the truth simply and factually. Even kids as young as three or four years of age are capable of understanding information if it is told to them in a simple, informative manner. Children have remarkable powers of imagination, and what they imagine is often far more devastating and difficult for them to handle than actual facts.

When discussing a chronic illness such as PD with young children, remember that these youngsters will take their cues from you. If you're upbeat and optimistic about the effects of the disease, they are likely to feel the same way. Saying, for instance, that "Grandpa has Parkinson's disease and may need to be in a wheelchair, but he can still take you to the zoo" rather than "Grandpa is very sick and he won't be able to play with you anymore" is far more positive and reassuring.

Be sure to explain any and all symptoms and side effects experienced by the patient, even if you think the child might not notice. If you have PD and depression is causing you to cry more often than usual, make sure that your children know that this is part of the disease and not related to anything they may have done. The more concrete the information is, the more the child will understand about the illness and about the parent's or grandparent's behavior.

It is important to give the child a chance to ask questions, not only at the time you tell them but throughout the course of the illness. Children may be particularly afraid of things you may not think they are old enough to even consider, such as if the disease is contagious or inherited. They should feel free to ask whatever is on their mind without being afraid of embarrassing or upsetting you.

Realize that your children will pass through many of the same stages of acceptance you will. They may become angry at you for no longer being the strong and omniscient provider. They will no doubt be afraid of losing you to complete disability or death. Many adult children are concerned about what their caregiver role should be: many fear losing their own, perhaps just recently gained, independence. In turn, they may feel guilty about resenting your illness and the demands it makes upon their lives.

Unfortunately, as a parent, it is up to you to recognize your children's emotions for what they are, and give them the room to experience them. Many patients find that family counseling, conducted by a reputable therapist, is the best way to deal with these issues in a supportive environment. Your physician or hospital social worker will be able to recommend a therapist if you so desire.

Getting Organized

"Everyone, including my doctor, told me to take things one day at a time," Alan says. "But I couldn't help it. Things just kept flying through my mind: Should I get a new doctor? Who can help me exercise properly? What will happen once I can't work? Put plainly and simply, I wanted to get organized."

Emotionally and physically, you're coming to terms with your disease. Nevertheless, a lifelong chronic illness will require a number of adjustments that may overwhelm you if you don't think and plan ahead. Make plans—and contingency plans—for your daily schedule. If you need daily care and your spouse is your major caregiver, decide what will happen if he or she is unable to help you for some reason. If you are still working, but have severe "off" times, decide now what you would do if you were suddenly incapacitated (most people, for instance, keep an extra dose of Sinemet with them at all times).

Luckily, you're not alone. Professionals and fellow patients are available to help you answer your myriad questions.

Tips for Telling People About PD:

1. Timing is important. If you wait too long, people may feel betrayed. If you tell a new acquaintance too soon, you may turn them off before they get a chance to know you. If you bring it up when you're distraught, you're likely to get a far different reaction from when you're in more control.
2. Decide whom you need to tell personally. If there are some people who should be told but don't need to hear it from you directly, ask a close friend or relative to tell them. If you're planning to tell co-workers, tell your supervisors first so they won't find out from someone else.
3. Try to anticipate how the person will react. You're better of not being caught completely off-guard by negative reactions. Self-help groups or counseling can help you sort out what the range of reactions may be.
4. Think about what you want or need from the person you're telling. Do you want time off from work? A shoulder to cry on? Help with chores? State your needs as clearly as you can; it will guide friends, relatives, and co-workers toward a positive reaction.
5. Guide people to sources of information. People may not want to burden you with questions or may be too confused or worried to ask. Bring educational materials with you from the APDA or elsewhere that may help.

   Accepting on an emotional level the fact that you or someone you love has a chronic illness is a never-ending process.

Getting to Know Your Health-Care Team

It is important for you to find professionals who specialize in Parkinson's disease or similar chronic illnesses. A local American Parkinson's Disease Information and Referral Center or other PD organization will be able to help you locate qualified personnel if your physician cannot. (Please see Appendix I for a list of referral centers.)

Neurologist: Many patients choose to have their primary-care physicians treat their Parkinson's disease as well, especially if other conditions, such as diabetes or heart disease, coexist. A regular visit—once or twice a year, maybe less—to a neurologist may help you and your primary physician get a more precise estimation of your particular stage of disease, perhaps refine your drug therapy, and gather information about new treatments. Your primary-care physician should have no objection to your seeing another doctor; in fact, he or she should encourage you to seek other opinions. It's important that each physician is kept apprised of your condition and course of treatment at all times.

Occupational Therapist (OT): This health-care professional is trained to assess your self-care skills, help you adapt to loss of motor skills, and, with the use of adaptive aids, maximize your independence. From cooking in the kitchen and feeding yourself, to speaking on the telephone or getting yourself in and out of the bathtub, the OT will help you to minimize the difficulties you may have in performing any of these or other tasks. You should seek the help of an OT when you are experiencing problems with activities of daily living, when you no longer enjoy some of the activities that used to give you pleasure, or if you start having falls or other accidents.

Physical Therapist: Since Parkinson's disease is a chronic illness affecting the mobility of every part of the body, physical therapy is essential for patients in all stages of the disease. A physical therapist, especially one trained in the special needs of PD patients, will help a PD patient maximize flexibility and posture through simple, painless stretching and strengthening exercises. In addition, physical therapists work with patients to achieve functional mobility, teaching them the easiest and safest ways to get in and out of bed, cook food and feed themselves, dress, bathe, and perform other daily activities that can become increasingly difficult as the disease progresses. Although physical therapy does not reverse or delay the symptoms of PD, it both helps patients make full use of their potential and prevents complications, particularly falls and fractures.

Speech Therapist: Parkinson's disease affects the speech and/or swallowing abilities of about 30 percent of PD patients. A speech therapist evaluates the communication status of the patient by looking at three components: language, speech, and oral movement. Like Beth, whom you met in the first chapter, many patients are first diagnosed because a spouse has noticed facial masking or slurring of words. The speech therapist teaches the family and patient about communication problems and ways to compensate for the affects of the disease.

Dietitian: Weight gain, weight loss, and protein redistribution are concerns for PD patients. A dietitian can evaluate the adequacy of your past dietary habits, recent weight changes, protein status, and the function of your gastrointestinal tract. After problems are identified, a dietitian will counsel you on ways to make sure you're getting a balanced diet. For those patients who have difficulty swallowing, the dietitian may consult with the speech and/or occupational therapist to help the patient deal with this problem.

Social Worker: Many hospitals and social service agencies have social workers to evaluate your psychosocial situation. Not every PD patient is lucky enough to have a spouse or supportive family, and often needs extra guidance in coping and adapting. The social worker also facilitates communication among patients, family, and involved medical personnel. Your physician may be able to suggest a hospital social worker who can determine the proper intervention such as individual or family counseling.

Financial Planner/Attorney: Attorneys specializing in wills and estate planning are crucial for someone facing a chronic, degenerative disease like PD. While a hospital social worker can help you deal with certain financial matters, a good financial attorney may be the best bet for you. See Chapter Nine for more information about your financial options and how to choose the best attorney for your needs.

Community Agencies: City and state Councils on the Elderly and other organizations provide a variety of services for senior adults, the disabled, the chronically ill, and caregivers. (For more information about these general resources, see both Chapter Nine and Appendix I.)

*   *   *

Your family and your friends will provide support as best they can to both you and your spouse. Nevertheless, two systems of support are especially crucial to you. First and foremost is your personal physician and his staff. You'll be visiting the doctor's office at least twice a year, perhaps more often. Another link to maintaining your health and good spirits is a network of people most PD patients say they couldn't do without: other PD patients and caregivers.

Your Primary Physician

Successful treatment of Parkinson's disease requires a partnership between you and your doctor, one that involves an honesty and openness you may not have with anyone else in your life. The variability of the course of the disease itself and the delicacy of its drug treatment demand an uncommonly intimate relationship between physician and patient.

In order for you to maintain your independence and enjoyment of life for as long as possible, you must feel free to tell your doctor the most private details of your life and bodily functions. You'll have to tell him when you're constipated, when you're sweating too much, when excessive drooling is upsetting your social life. You'll talk about your sex life and how the disease and the medication used to treat it have affected it. If you hallucinate or feel depressed, if you're suddenly freezing in the middle of your morning walk, your doctor must know about it. Otherwise, you will continue to suffer in silence.

Needless to say, you must trust and, to a certain extent, like your primary physician. This isn't to say that the two of you will become bosom buddies; your doctor must keep a certain professional distance to provide you with the best, most objective care. What it does mean, however, is that you have to feel comfortable with your doctor, and he or she with you, since the relationship between you may last for several years, perhaps a lifetime.

Communication is not the only issue to consider when evaluating your physician. Does he or she have a practice that specializes in Parkinson's disease or at least treat a number of PD patients? Does he or she keep up-to-date on current therapies and medical advances? If you're unsure about your doctor's qualifications, you can check with your local medical society or with your local American Parkinson's Disease Information and Referral Center (see Appendix I).

If for any reason you are not happy with your current physician, you should feel free to choose another. This should not, of course, be done lightly, especially if your doctor has been caring for you and your family for a long time. On the other hand, since your medical therapy may require complex and constant adjustments, your physician should be as well versed in PD and as open to your needs as possible.

Establishing Good Doctor-Patient Relationships

In order to maintain the best relationship possible with your doctor and his or her staff, the following procedures are recommended:

1. *Manage minor health complaints at home*: Unfortunately, having Parkinson's disease does not make you immune to the common flu or cold. Although your first instinct may be to phone the doctor, these problems usually resolve themselves within a few days without medical treatment. Safe and reliable medications for symptomatic relief are available for common illness management without necessitating a costly and inconvenient trip to your doctor's office.
2. *Use your doctor's telephone services intelligently*:
   - Let the office nurse help decide if your problem warrants a visit.
   - The patient, not the caregiver, should describe symptoms to the doctor or nurse. Relaying symptoms or advice through a third person significantly increases the odds of miscommunication.
   - Have the phone number of your pharmacy available.
   - Know the names and dosages of the drugs you take regularly.
   - PROTEST if your call is not returned in a reasonable amount of time (within a few hours or a day depending on the urgency of your concern).
3. Inquire if routine laboratory or health screening tests (blood pressure readings, for example) can be done without the additional expense and time involved in an office visit.

The Well-Stocked Medicine Cabinet

Medications/Products

Acetaminophen: for fever and pain; not anti-inflammatory

Aspirin: for fever and pain

Calamine lotion: to reduce itching and to dry poison ivy rashes

Benadryl 25 mg: antihistamine (for runny noses, rashes, allergic rashes or hives, beestings), antinausea/motion-sickness, antitussive (cough reliever); also helps reduce tremor

Dextromethorphan cough suppressant: available in many over-the-counter cough medications

Zinc ointment: soothing, water-resistant, ultimate sunscreen

Mild soap: best for sensitive skin

Bucladin-S: prescription drug for nausea and vomiting

Equalactin: bowel regulator; helps *both* diarrhea and constipation

Hydrocortisone cream: topical anti-inflammatory agent, 1% solution needs prescription, 0.5% over-the-counter

Hydrogen peroxide: best general antiseptic

Ibuprofen 200 mg: stronger pain reliever than aspirin or acetaminophen

Ipecac syrup: to induce vomiting in case of poisoning; call local poison control center *prior* to administering

K-Y jelly: water-soluble lubricant, safe for use in vaginal area

Liquid antacid: use as needed after meals to deal with hyperacidity; inform physician if chronic problem

Moisturizers with urea and/or lactic acid (SeaBreeze cream, Aquacare, Betamide are good brands; equal to more expensive brands)

Polysporin ointment or triple-antibiotic ointment if not allergic to neomycin; good for topical applications to superficial skin infections

Suntan lotion containing PABA: minimum of SPF 8 to offer protection even for dark skin

Vaseline: general water-resistant lubricant

Supplies/Equipment

Vaporizer—a cool mist setting is best

Thermometer

Package of small needles/TB syringes provide "handle" to remove splinters, etc.

Magnifying glass

Tapered-point tweezers

1" Band-Aid strips

Small, sharp-point scissors

Kling-type stretch gauze roll

Ace or other elastic bandage (3" most versatile)

Hot-water bottle (can be used in place of heating pad)

"Blue ice" disposable pack or heavy Ziploc small freezer bags filled with ice

Good penlight

Plastic or silk tape (1"), nonadhesive

Box of toddler-size disposable diapers to use as large wound or pressure dressing

TO BE AVOIDED

Laxatives

Feminine hygiene sprays, douches, etc.

Skin scrubs or harsh cloths (could break small blood vessels)

Over-the-counter sleep inducers

Over-the-counter diet pills

Aerosol sprays

4. Schedule appointments midweek, early in the doctor's morning or afternoon schedule. Arrive on time, and remind the receptionist of your presence if you are still in the waiting room 30 minutes after your scheduled appointment.

5. Take a concerned person with you to hear the doctor's evaluation, and perhaps make some notes for future reference. However, communicate directly with your physician and don't expect your spouse or caregiver to do the talking for both of you.

Caregivers, bring a notebook that lists your questions and

in which you can write down the doctor's recommendations. Remember to be respectful of the patient during the interview. Although you may need to contradict or add to his or her version of events, try to do this as gently as possible. If you are going to be the one to administer medicine or physical therapy, be sure to ask for explanations and clarifications of instructions at this time.

6. Tell your doctor the WHOLE truth; withholding facts for fear of embarrassment can easily lead to misdiagnosis or unnecessary treatment. Let your doctor know if you do not understand his terminology. Restate his assessment and treatment recommendations in your own language to ensure good communication.

7. Cultivate a close relationship with the doctor's nurse. In most practices, the nurse is the person who will talk with you by phone in between visits and who can teach your family about specific care issues. Help the nurse to remember your family and track your concerns.

A Network of Hope

Both the physical and emotional issues related to Parkinson's disease make it all too easy for a patient and family to withdraw from the world—so many physical limitations to overcome, so many potentially embarrassing situations (such as falling or tremoring or drooling) you may feel you must avoid, so much frustration and sorrow to experience. Stepping back out into the world may be one of the toughest things to do.

Luckily, there are about a million people out there who know just what you're feeling. They want to help you deal with the many problems you face, and they can do it with firsthand knowledge that even the best health-care professionals lack. They are your fellow PD patients and they form a warm and loving network of support.

Today, about one million Americans suffer from Parkinson's disease. Many of these patients and families belong to one of the hundreds of Parkinson's disease support groups located in cities and towns throughout the country. Most of these support groups are organized with the help of local hospitals and are linked to the American Parkinson's Disease Association.

Support groups meet on a regular basis, usually once a month, to discuss common problems, form friendships, and learn coping strategies from both professional guest speakers and fellow sufferers. One function of a support group is to disseminate helpful information through newsletters, guest speakers, open meetings, health fairs, and symposia. Support groups learn about community resources and networking strategies. Many support groups offer their own exercise and/or speech therapy sessions; others establish respite or adult care centers. Some groups have published books and sponsored videotapes of their own.

You may think you're the only person in the world who suddenly freezes in the middle of a step or who is embarrassed by tremor. If you join a support group, you'll find other men and women who experience the same symptoms and side effects that trouble you.

Perhaps the most important role of a support group is that of friend and willing listener. No matter how understanding your co-workers and friends may be about your PD, you don't want to burden them with your problems or overwhelm them with your enthusiasm over a medical treatment. In addition, you may have discovered, through your illness, a new sense of purpose, hope, and direction. A support group will provide you with a nurturing and understanding environment in which to explore these newfound feelings. Take advantage of this most important resource. (For more information, please see Appendix I.)

Do you have trouble getting in and out of the bathtub? Are you plagued by aches and pains? Do you worry that you shouldn't be driving your car anymore? In Chapter Seven, The A to Z Guide to Symptoms and Side Effects, these issues and others will be addressed in an accessible encyclopedic format. Just look through the Symptoms and Side Effects Index (on page 118) to find some possible solutions to your particular problems.

Chapter Seven

The A to Z Guide to Symptoms and Side Effects

As you've learned, neurochemistry is a complex and interrelated system. Parkinson's disease involves a depletion of dopamine, a powerful neurotransmitter. When your brain lacks dopamine, it cannot send the appropriate messages about movement to the body's muscles. As a result, you suffer from rigidity, tremor, bradykinesia, and other symptoms of this chemical imbalance.

In attempting to replace dopamine or otherwise stimulate dopamine receptors, we risk disturbing other systems within the brain, thereby causing side effects. All of the drugs used to treat Parkinson's disease have the potential to cause a number of unpleasant side effects.

Is it important to learn the difference between symptoms of the disease process itself and the side effects of the drugs you take? For some of the more minor complaints, probably not, especially since both the disease and anti-PD drugs may cause the same problems. Some patients will become constipated due to the disease process itself, for instance, while others are affected by constipation only by using certain anti-Parkinson drugs; still others react to both. Only by trial and error will the cause of such complaints be discovered.

You should, however, learn to distinguish between what happens when you take too much medicine and what happens when you take too little. The drugs used to treat PD may often *overstimulate* the dopamine circuit in the brain. A steady overdose of PD drugs causes certain side effects that many patients mistakenly assume to be symptoms of the disease. Among them are dyskinesias (involuntary movements), hallucinations, and dystonias (abnormal, often painful, postures).

This guide will help you monitor and control both the symptoms and the side effects of Parkinson's disease. In addition, some of the most pressing issues facing PD patients, including employment and hospitalization, are covered here as well. Read through the whole guide or look through the list above to find the topic that most concerns you at this moment. As your doctor's partner, it's up to you to keep track of your medical condition between visits and help him devise a treatment strategy that works best for you.

Aches and Pains

"I believe that my very first symptom of the disease was a kind of deep achiness that sort of wandered," reports Ruth, a 70-year-old woman who was diagnosed about three years ago. "One day it would be in my legs, another time in my hands and lower arms. I still feel it often." Although PD has often been described as a painless illness, many patients—up to 30 percent according to some studies—do in fact complain of achiness, numbness, and fatigue. Others describe it as tingling or tightness.

Most aches and pains experienced by PD patients stem from the muscular rigidity caused by the disease. Rigid muscles are in a state of constant tension. They become sore from the effort of maintaining this tension and also from holding your body in abnormal positions. Persistent lower back pain, for instance, often results from the stooped posture common to many PD patients. Tenting of the hands, consistently leaning to one side, and turning your feet inward, all may cause localized achiness.

Severe muscular rigidity also manifests itself as cramping (see Dystonia). Many patients are plagued with leg cramps during the night. Others find that their feet cramp up during or after exercise and their hands spasm if they write for a long time.

Some patients describe sensations of heat and cold in the limbs. Sometimes a patient will complain about feet or hands that are freezing, although no measurable difference in skin temperature can be detected even by a physician. Feelings of external warmth—even burning—of the hands and feet are also common, and may be accompanied by flushing of the skin. Why such sensory changes are experienced by some patients is not fully understood.

Treatment: For general relief from achiness, warm baths and full body massages should help to relax muscles and increase comfort. Unfortunately, aspirin and other analgesics do not seem to ease PD pain, but stretching exercises, such as the ones described in Chapter Five, will go a long way in helping relieve your stiffness and soreness. If you suffer from leg, foot, or hand cramping, you should massage the affected limb gently, then apply heat with either a hot-water bottle or heating pad.

In general, the best way to treat temperature fluctuations is to do whatever feels comfortable: wear woolen socks if your feet are cold, dunk your hands in cold water if it helps stop the burning sensation. If any of these sensory disturbances cause you severe pain, please speak with your physician. Medication adjustments may be required or a cause other than PD may be responsible.

Bathing and Bathroom Organization

It has become something of a cliche to say that more accidents happen in our bathrooms than on our highways, but it's a fact of life, especially for the parkinsonian plagued with stiffness and balance problems.

All bathroom surfaces, from the floor to the toilet to a glass shower door, are extremely hard and also have a tendency to become slippery. If you have any trouble with your balance, walking, or transferring (getting into and out of the tub or on and off the toilet), you can make your bathroom safer by removing as much glass as possible. Trade glass shower partitions for cloth or plastic curtains. Replace drinking glasses with paper or plastic cups.

Next, remove scatter rugs and nonrubberized bath mats, and if possible, put down wall-to-wall bathroom carpeting. This will keep the floor, even if wet, from becoming slippery and will alleviate the need for mats. If carpeting is not an option, put nonskid material around the sink, toilet, and tub. If you haven't done so already, put some in the tub and shower themselves.

If you're at all unsteady, install grab bars around the tub and toilet. That way, if you feel as if you're going to fall, you won't grab either a towel rack or shower curtain, both of which are apt to come tumbling down and take you with them.

Grab bars will also help you get around the bathroom more easily, providing support as you walk and leverage for transfers. Some toilet seats are quite low to the floor, making transfers more difficult. Some patients find that raised toilet seats, which can be purchased from any medical supply store, provide easier access.

For many patients, nothing soothes sore muscles or stressed nerves more than a hot bath. Unfortunately, getting in and out of a tub—especially an old-fashioned standing type—can prove to be quite a chore. Grab bars will help; so will the aid of a caregiver. When all else fails, a hot shower is a soothing compromise.

To shower safely, some patients find sitting on a stool in the shower both comfortable and convenient. Use of a handheld shower nozzle allows you to wash more thoroughly with limited bending and stretching. Often slippery and uncooperative, washcloths and soap bars can be replaced by soap-on-a-rope, bath mitts, or a homemade all-in-one bathing aid: take a large loofah or soft sponge, make a slit in its center, then place a bar of soap inside.

Once out of the tub or shower, slip into a luxurious terry cloth robe and pat yourself dry. This may help you avoid twisting and turning to get at the hard-to-reach places. On the other hand, your muscles should be relaxed after a hot bath or shower and you may want to use this opportunity to do some stretching while drying (preferably in a safe area in case you should fall)! (For tips about performing other bathroom chores see Dental Care.)

Bed Mobility

Most PD patients have difficulty sleeping at one time or another. Most sleep problems are related to drug therapy or to poor sleep habits. (See Sleep Disorders.) Some, however, are related to the ways in which bradykinesia and rigidity interfere with getting into and out of bed, turning over, and otherwise changing positions in bed.

To make your bedroom safe and comfortable, first remove all throw rugs from around the bed itself and from the major passage routes into and out of the room. Install nightlights so that nocturnal trips to the bathroom or kitchen are safe. Light switches should be easily reachable; many patients find a switch on a cord next to the bed convenient.

If you need help getting in and out of bed, bed rails, at least on one side of the bed, can help; they also make good grab bars to help you move from side to side in bed. Another adaptive aid is the overhead trapeze, which can further aid in self-mobility. Or you could position a sturdy nightstand in such a way that it doubles as a balancing support, both for transfers and to grip as you turn over.

Satin sheets or pajamas are other helpful bedtime aids. Because they're so slippery, they make moving around in bed much easier.

Be careful, however, not to overdose on satin: Your bed can become so slippery that you'll fall right out! Choose either pajamas *or* sheets. If that's still too slippery, you might try sewing a large square of satin or other silky material at the center of the bed so that you'll have traction for your feet, arms, and head. Other people find that top-quality cotton sheets (200-thread-count, for example) are smooth enough to facilitate movement.

Even with your way paved with satin, turning over and getting in and out of bed may be difficult for you. Here are some physical therapy tips that should help you:

- To roll over: Most patients have one direction in which they roll more easily; try to use your best side when moving about in bed. When you're trying to turn onto your side from a flat position, first push off with the opposite foot (if you're trying to roll onto your right side, push off with your left foot), lean toward the left first with the hips, then the trunk, then finally the shoulders and arms. To get a little extra momentum, swing your arms a few times in the direction of the roll. That should get you onto your right side.
- To sit up: First, roll onto your best side. Then push down on the bed with your arms at chest level and, at the same time, swing your legs over the edge of the bed.
- To get out of bed: Take your time. Many patients feel a bit dizzy when they first sit up from a supine position. Start when you feel comfortable, then, with both feet flat on the floor and your hands beside your hips, gently push yourself into a standing posture. Use the springiness of the mattress to give you a little push by bouncing a bit before pushing off with your hands.

Other bedroom hints:

- Use a comforter both as a bedspread and a blanket. It is both lightweight and warm. An electric blanket provides a steady, even heat over your entire body, which may help keep you from trying to toss and turn in search of a "warm spot."
- Use a blanket lift to keep blankets off your feet at night if they restrict your mobility; but wear socks to keep your feet warm.

- Keep all necessities (glasses, false teeth, alarm clock, reading material) next to you on a sturdy night table. If you use the night table as a physical therapy tool, be sure to put everything in a drawer.
- If you need to urinate often during the night, consider moving your bed (or bedroom) closer to the bathroom if necessary, or place a portable commode near the bed.
- If you have a spouse or partner who sleeps with you, keep in mind that your partner may be disturbed by your movements or discomfort. Some couples opt for twin beds if the disruption becomes problematic for either partner.

Constipation

Perhaps the most universal of all PD complaints is constipation. Why does it affect so many patients? One reason is that both the disease process itself *and* PD drug therapy cause the action of the intestines to slow down. In addition, many PD patients reduce both their activity level (because of muscular rigidity and bradykinesia) and their fiber in-take (if they ever were eating enough fiber, they may now have difficulty chewing and swallowing fiber-rich foods), thereby further slowing the passage of stool through the large intestine.

Another factor is the difficulty of the act of defecation itself. All the muscles of the rectum and abdominal wall are involved in ridding our bodies of waste. Unfortunately, these same muscles may be affected by PD's rigidity and bradykinesia.

In addition, drugs used to treat these symptoms may also affect our digestive tract. As you may remember from Chapter Four, anticholinergic drugs were first used to treat stomach upsets by slowing down muscular activity in the stomach and intestines. It should come as no surprise, then, that the use of these drugs—although very effective in reducing tremor and other symptoms—may aggravate constipation as well.

Treatment: By itself, constipation is not a cause for concern. Contrary to popular belief, there is no medical necessity to move the bowels every day; you won't "poison" your body if you do not defecate every day or even every few days. However, you may feel bloated and uncomfortable (many patients complain of head-aches when they are constipated) after a day or two without moving your bowels.

To keep your intestinal tract functioning as well as possible:

- Drink at least eight 8-ounce glasses of water every day (but drink most of your water during the morning and early afternoon so that you won't have to get up in the night to urinate).
- Exercise regularly. This will help stretch and strengthen the abdominal and pelvic muscles needed in the act of defecation. Walking also helps propel the stool into the lower intestine.
- Some patients set a specific time of the day to move their bowels (perhaps in the morning after a warm drink), giving themselves plenty of time to relax into the task.
- Eat plenty of fresh fruit and vegetables, including the trusty home remedy of figs and prunes.
- Gradually add more fiber to your diet by adding a cup of un-processed bran cereal (20 grams of fiber) or taking up to six tablespoons of coarse bran per day (3 tablespoons at each meal). Sprinkle the bran into applesauce, onto cereal, or mix into yogurt. Be sure to increase the amount of fiber in your diet slowly, otherwise you may feel bloated or suffer from excess stomach gas.
- When moving the bowels, sit comfortably on a toilet with knees drawn up to help the abdominal muscles pass the stool. If you have grab bars around the toilet, use them for extra leverage if necessary. Don't strain too hard, or you'll risk developing hemorrhoids.

Keep in mind that it's far easier to prevent constipation than to treat it. Long-term use of laxatives is most destructive, and can lead to a total loss of muscle tone, resulting in chronic impactions. If a laxative must be used for brief period, a mild agent such as milk of magnesia should be selected. Glycerin suppositories can ease the passage of hard stools, and stool softeners such as Colace may be used on a daily basis if dietary measures alone are ineffective. (Please note: Mineral-oil preparations should NOT be used as laxatives if the patient has trouble swallowing because aspiration—breathing in—of these substances can lead to pneumonia.)

Dementia

Some patients experience temporary confusion, hallucinations, and/or loss of memory at some point during the course of their disease while on drug therapy. Some of these disturbances are related to the aging process; as we get older, brain cells die and patches of memory and thinking processes are lost. This condition is usually quite mild. Other mental changes experienced by the PD patient are related to the amount of medication and the length of time the patient has been taking it. (See Hallucinations.)

Other patients, however, exhibit a more serious decline in memory, thinking, and behavior called dementia. Researchers estimate that approximately 30 percent of all PD patients, especially those over 70 years of age, have some degree of dementia, but whether it is directly related to PD is unknown. Parkinson's disease and Alzheimer's disease—a common form of dementia—affect the same population, namely the elderly, and it is quite possible that the two conditions may coexist in the same patient.

Treatment: Treating dementia associated with PD is quite frustrating and difficult. The drugs used to treat the motor symptoms of PD may exacerbate dementia, forcing patients to accept decreased mobility and increased tremor in order to alleviate the dementia. If dementia is not anti-Parkinson drug-related, then little can be done to treat it. A visit to a neurologist is advisable to rule out any other causes and to gauge the severity of the patient's condition.

Dementia often takes its greatest toll on the caregivers and other family members who must watch their loved one steadily lose the ability to think, remember, and behave in a rational manner. If you are a caregiver, safety becomes a major concern, since the patient may act in ways dangerous to himself and to others: forgetting to turn off a stove burner, leaving a lighted cigarette somewhere, ignoring instructions to take medication. From helping the patient dress and use the bathroom, to cooking meals, to dealing with often irrational behavior, a caregiver's days and nights n endless. It is essential that you care for yourself as well e patient. Get help from family members or city/state Read Chapter Eight for more details.

Dental Care

As you age, caring for your teeth and gums becomes more important. First, your gums naturally recede as you age, which may cause your teeth to shift and/or decay more easily. Second, many elderly people have difficulty chewing hard foods, which is one of the best natural ways to stimulate gums and keep teeth healthy. Add Parkinson's disease to the aging process and you may have dental disaster if you're not careful.

Not only will your disease add to your disinclination to eat chewy or hard foods, but many anti-Parkinson drugs cause dry mouth. A lack of saliva makes your teeth more vulnerable to decay. In addition, many parkinsonians grind their teeth and clench their jaws, perhaps due to increased tremor and/or rigidity. Such friction and tension can damage tooth enamel and/or result in broken or chipped teeth. (Constant jaw clenching can even cause tension headaches.)

For the PD patient, a healthy mouth is especially important. Having all of your teeth will allow you to speak more clearly, help your face to look younger and more responsive, and allow you to chew and swallow your foods properly.

Treatment: Firm toothbrushes are best for removing plaque and debris from your teeth and gums. Many patients opt for a toothbrush with firm bristles in the middle and soft ones on the outside, so that the gums are not overly stimulated. Although many of us were taught to brush in an up-and-down direction, a circular motion will clean the teeth and gums more efficiently. Use a fluoride toothpaste and/or oral rinse at least twice a day to help prevent decay exacerbated by your medication. Flossing between the teeth and up into the gums, although time-consuming, is the best form of gum disease prevention known. If possible, floss every day.

If decreased grip and hand strength make it difficult for you to use an ordinary toothbrush, special brushes with larger handles are available at some medical supply stores. You can also make the handle of your own toothbrush larger by inserting a rubber bicycle handle on the end or by punching holes through a tennis ball and inserting the toothbrush through it. As for flossing, ask your pharmacist to recommend a sturdy dental floss holder and/or floss threader to make your chore easier. If these measures fail, try using an electric toothbrush, which does most of the work for you, or a device called Interplak, which acts as both a toothbrush and a flosser.

If you find yourself grinding your teeth or clenching your jaw—particularly when you sleep (your spouse may be able to tell you if you do)—you may need a protective mouthpiece to preserve and protect your teeth. Ask your dentist or physician to recommend one to you.

Depression

For some patients, overwhelming feelings of sadness and a lack of energy are the first symptoms of Parkinson's disease, even before a diagnosis is made. For others, these feelings emerge much later, when their state of disability is at its peak. Depression may occur and recur several times during the course of the disease and may last from a few weeks to many months.

Depression is more than lingering unhappiness; it is prolonged and leads to a disruption of one's lifestyle and activities. Depression involves a pervasive sense of pessimism: Not only are things bad now but they will be bad forever. No external circumstance, such as a visit from good friends or a vacation, will lift someone who is clinically depressed from a state of gloom and sadness. Second, these feelings are accompanied by physical changes: Sleep patterns will shift, with patients sleeping far more or less than usual. Appetite, too, either diminishes or grows to an abnormal degree. Patients who are depressed withdraw from normal activities, even the ones that once gave them the most pleasure. Feeling that life is no longer worth living, some depressed patients turn to thoughts of suicide. Some end their own lives.

In many instances, depression has no identifiable cause. In others, it may be triggered by a sad event, such as a death or loss of a job. Chronic illness is a major cause of depression among people of all age groups. Some research indicates that as many as 30–40 percent of the chronically ill will experience periods of depression, compared with about 10 percent among the general population. Among PD patients, the percentage is even higher, affecting more

Signs and Symptoms of Depression

Poor appetite
Weight loss
Sleep disturbances (insomnia or excessive sleep)
Low energy
Loss of sex drive
Feelings of extreme sadness, anxiousness, and worry
Loss of interest or pleasure in usual activities
Poor concentration
Thoughts of suicide

than 50 percent of all parkinsonians at some point in the course of their disease. Scientists have examined the possibility that the disease process itself is to blame, at least in part. As discussed in Chapter Two, the neurotransmitters involved in movement are also related to other processes in the brain, including those that control certain emotions and moods. Norepinephrine and serotonin, known to be depleted in the brains of depressed individuals, are also found in lesser amounts in the brain of the PD patient.

In addition, of course, are the emotional strains on a person suffering from a degenerative brain disease such as PD. Low self-esteem, fear of dependence, and negative, often embarrassing physical changes such as tremor and stooped posture can lead to overwhelming feelings of helplessness and despondency. Guilt over being a burden to one's spouse and/or other family members, depression over the loss of employment, and fear of financial restrictions are other stressors on the emotional stability of a parkinsonian.

Treatment: The first step in treating depression is for the patient, family, and the physician to recognize and admit the problem together. Not everyone who is depressed cries or expresses feelings of sadness. Instead, the patient may be irritable, angry, or simply withdrawn. Indeed, often patients themselves are unaware that they are depressed. Caregivers should be on the lookout for the symptoms listed in the box above and alert the physician if the condition persists.

Every patient will experience depression in a different way and respond to different therapies. Many patients snap themselves out of their blue mood by getting involved in a support group, exercising on a regular basis, or starting a new project. In other cases, psychotherapy may be warranted, especially if feelings of low self-esteem and lack of self-confidence do not allow the patient to venture out into the world.

If you are depressed, regaining an interest in the world around you, rather than focusing on your disability, is the key to renewed emotional health. If you lack energy and motivation, set yourself small, easy-to-achieve goals. Exercise for 15 minutes today. Start a new sewing or other project this week. Meet two new people at this month's support group meeting. Every time you reach a goal, congratulate yourself and take some time to feel good about what you've accomplished. Slowly but surely, your self-esteem will grow and your activities will once again give you pleasure.

If you still can't get yourself out of your blue mood, you may want to seek the help of a psychotherapist. He or she may be able to help you locate the root causes of your depression, some of which may be unrelated to your disease, and work through your feelings with you. If your spouse and other family members are adversely affected by your disease and/or your depression, you may want to consult a family therapist together.

Your doctor may also prescribe a drug to treat your depression. Antidepressants fall into two general categories: tricyclic antidepressants and monoamine oxidase inhibitors. PD patients should avoid the MAO inhibitors used to treat depression. These MAO inhibitors, unlike selegiline, block both MAO A and MAO B and may cause unpleasant side effects. Tricyclic antidepressants, on the other hand, are safe for most PD patients. Nortriptyline, also known as Pamelor or Aventyl, and amitriptyline, also known as Elavil, are often prescribed to PD patients, especially those who also feel anxious or who have trouble sleeping since they also work as mild sedatives. Imipramine (Tofranil) is another tricyclic antidepressant; it is less sedating and may be best for patients who do not respond to nortriptyline or amitriptyline. Fluoxitine (Prozac) may also be used.

Be aware that although antidepressants may elevate your mood, they may also cause side effects similar to those caused by your anti-Parkinson medication. Dry mouth, constipation, urinary tract dysfunction, loss of libido, and blurred vision are some of the most common antidepressant side effects.

In very rare cases when both psychotherapy and antidepressant drug therapy fail, ECT (electroconvulsive or electroshock therapy) should be considered if the depression is severe. It is a decision to be made jointly among doctor, patient, and family.

Dizziness

Approximately 20 to 25 percent of all patients treated with Sinemet or other anti-Parkinson drugs experience some degree of what is known as orthostatic hypotension, which simply means that your blood pressure drops when you stand up. Although not dangerous in and of itself, this drop in blood pressure may make you feel dizzy, lose your balance, and injure yourself in a fall.

How does PD cause orthostatic hypotension? As you may remember from Chapter Two, dopamine also works outside the brain. One system it affects controls the body's temperature and blood pressure. In a healthy body, this system works automatically to keep the blood pressure and temperature steady, much the way an automobile's cruise control regulates the speed of your car. Cruise control keeps your car running at 55 miles an hour even if you're driving up a hill; your blood pressure is regulated by certain systems to remain steady whether you sit down, stand up, or lie down. However, an increase of dopamine in the body can put your body's cruise control system out of whack, resulting in a precipitous drop in blood pressure when you stand up.

In addition, lack of exercise and the tendency to remain seated over long periods of time result in poor circulation. Blood pools in the lower extremities rather than flowing as quickly and evenly as it should into the upper body and brain. When you stand, your brain does not receive the blood it needs and dizziness may result.

Treatment: If you suffer from periodic or constant low blood pressure, your doctor will probably adjust your medication. Smaller doses of levodopa and/or anticholinergics may be required to bring blood pressure under control. Exercise will keep the blood circulating more evenly. In addition, you might want to try wearing support hose to keep the blood from pooling in the legs.

Dressing

Dressing can be both tiring and time-consuming for patients who have lost the fine motor skills necessary for buttoning and zipping clothes or the muscular coordination necessary for putting on pants and jackets. Nevertheless, most patients feel more comfortable dressing themselves, even if it takes longer than it might with help from others.

Luckily, there is a wide variety of easy-to-wear, stylish fashions that avoid complicated closures. Sweatsuits, with their pullover tops, elastic waistband pants, and bright colors, are perfect for the PD patient with a casual lifestyle. So long as they are clean and color coordinated, sweatsuits can be worn almost everywhere—to the movies, restaurants, and shopping.

Velcro is a PD patient's best friend. A clever tailor can adapt all items of clothing with this type of closure, avoiding the need for zippers and buttons. Many shoes are now outfitted with Velcro, eliminating shoelaces altogether; if you have a favorite pair of tie shoes, a shoemaker may be able to adapt them with either Velcro closures or elastic shoelaces.

In addition, there are a number of adaptive aids available at certain medical supply stores and through catalogues (see Appendix I) that will make dressing easier for you. A dressing stick is useful for pulling trousers and underclothing over your feet and legs. You can also use it to reach for clothes located near you. A button hook slips through the button hole and pulls the button back through it. Other tips for safe and easy dressing include:

- If one side is stiffer than the other, put on and take off clothes from the stiff side first so that your mobility is increased.
- If your balance is affected, do not try to dress standing up. Instead, sit on the edge of bed or on a chair to dress.
- Choose clothing that closes in the front; reaching behind to zipper or button is difficult for everyone, with PD or without.
- Put on your shoes with a long-handled shoehorn.
- Lower clothes rods in closets so you don't have to reach too high for items.
- Lay out your clothes in the order in which you'll put them on and place them on a chair or bed near you.

If you continue to have trouble dressing, you may want to seek the help of an occupational therapist who has experience with PD patients.

Driving

If you were a good driver before your diagnosis, you're likely to remain a good driver for years to come, unless your disease progresses quite rapidly. Unfortunately, your limited mobility may diminish your driving skills at some point. Moving your foot back and forth from the brake pedal to the gas pedal may be slowed considerably. You may not be able to turn your head from side to side quickly or look out the back windshield. In addition, the medications you take to alleviate PD symptoms may make you sleepy from time to time, which certainly affects your driving skills. Once your reaction time and line of vision are so hampered, driving becomes hazardous. If you have any question about your driving ability, attend a driving school to have your skills assessed by professionals.

Giving up your driving privileges may be very difficult for you, since it will diminish your independence to some degree. Remember, though, that nothing is more important than your safety and the safety of others. If you do give up driving, you'll soon find many other transportation options: public buses or subways, taxicabs, willing friends and relatives. Accept these options cheerfully and use them often; do not let your inability to drive isolate you from your favorite activities.

Drooling

Otherwise known as sialorrhea, drooling is one of the more embarrassing but treatable symptoms of Parkinson's disease. Contrary to what you may think, Parkinson's disease does not cause you to produce more saliva. The problem comes instead from the fact that your swallowing reflex has been diminished due to bradykinesia; therefore, saliva collects in the mouth instead of being swallowed. If enough collects, it slips out of your mouth and you drool.

Treatment: Many anti-Parkinson drugs result in both improved swallowing and a lessening of saliva production. In fact, many patients end up suffering from dry mouth (see below) instead. Nevertheless, drooling remains a problem for some, especially in the later stages of disease.

If you have trouble with drooling, remember that because of your disease, you cannot rely on *automatically* swallowing. Instead, you must force yourself to *remember to swallow.* Sucking on a piece of hard candy or chewing gum helps a great deal. This method won't help at night, however, when many patients suffer from sialorrhea most. If you collect a lot of saliva in the back of the throat at night, try sleeping on your side so you don't wake yourself up choking.

If drooling becomes unresponsive to medications your doctor may prescribe, it is essential for caregivers to make sure the patient doesn't choke by using a bulb syringe to remove the pooled saliva. Family members may feel more secure if they receive training in first aid and the Heimlich maneuver (see the accompanying box). Classes on these subjects are also available from the American Red Cross or American Heart Association.

Dry Mouth

Ironically, many PD patients suffer from two quite opposite complaints, drooling (see above) and dry mouth. A lack of saliva is caused by many anti-Parkinson drugs, especially anticholinergics. It is exacerbated by stress, smoking, and the aging process.

In addition to causing discomfort, dry mouth is also unsanitary and potentially harmful to your teeth and digestion. Saliva prepares food for swallowing and begins the breakdown of food for absorption farther along the digestive tract (see "Swallowing" under Eating). Saliva also contains immune substances that help to protect the teeth, gums, and soft tissues of the mouth from attack by bacteria and fungi. Bad breath is an unpleasant side effect of dry mouth, as are cracked lips and burning sensations of the gums and tongue.

Treatment: Water, and lots of it, is one of the best treatments for dry mouth. Always drink water while you eat, which will also help

The Heimlich Maneuver
For the Choking Victim

The ability to swallow properly is often lost to PD patients, especially in the later stages of disease.

The victim should be sitting or standing.

1. Grasp the victim from behind with your hands around his/her waist.
2. Make a fist with one hand and place it, thumb side inward, on the victim's abdomen, midway between the waist and the rib cage.
3. Grasp your fist with your other hand and thrust forcefully inward and upward. Each new thrust should be a separate and distinct movement.

Repeat until the food is dislodged from the throat.

If the victim is especially obese or is pregnant, it is safer and easier to perform a chest thrust. The same two-hand technique is used, but grasp the victim at the breastbone (a little higher up directly under the breasts) rather than at the abdomen.

you avoid choking on food. In addition, you might try keeping a thermos of water near you all day, taking sips whenever you feel dry. This way, you'll get your recommended 6–8 glasses of water every day easily. Suck on sugar-free candies or chew sugarless gum to help stimulate the production of saliva. If your mouth is particularly parched and sore, try coating it with cocoa butter or olive oil.

Limit the amount of coffee, diet sodas, citrus fruit juices, and liquor you drink, for they can both dehydrate the body and irritate the mouth.

Dyskinesia

"It's as if I weren't my own pilot anymore," Caspar, the 76-year-old patient who's suffered with PD for more than fifteen years, describes. "I sit or stand there wriggling like I'm dancing. And no matter how hard I try, I can't stop." If you've been taking Sinemet for more than two or three years, it's likely you've already had experiences similar to Caspar's.

Involuntary or abnormal movement, also known as dyskinesia or chorea, is the most common and disruptive side effect of long-term anti-Parkinson medication. Such movements include everything from barely discernible twitches and jerks to disruptive twisting or writhing movements. They can involve any and all parts of the body.

Ironically, dyskinesias are usually caused by an *overdose* of dopamine in your striatum. At some point in the course of drug treatment, your brain may become hypersensitive to levodopa therapy. Even small amounts of the drug will cause side effects like dyskinesia. Or you may become resistant to Sinemet and need higher doses of the drug to alleviate your symptoms. In either case, your brain receives more dopamine than it can handle at certain points during the day. Some patients suffer from dyskinesias for just five to ten minutes when their medication first kicks in; others experience peak-dose dyskinesia about an hour or so into a dose; others feel dyskinetic as their dose wears off. As drug therapy continues and the disease progresses, a certain amount of dyskinetic action can last all day.

Dyskinetic movements are rarely dangerous to your health; only when they disrupt your balance, causing you to fall, do they present a hazard. Nevertheless, they are both embarrassing and uncomfortable. Many patients prefer to limit their activities, especially eating and walking, during the times when dyskinesia is most likely to occur.

Treatment: Unfortunately, the only treatment currently available for dyskinesia is a reduction in levodopa therapy, which may increase your parkinsonism. Your doctor may decide to decrease your daily dose of Sinemet and add a dopamine agonist, such as bromocriptine or pergolide. Agonists stimulate the dopamine receptors directly, bypassing the need for dopamine itself.

Dystonia

A tented hand, a turned-in foot, a twisted trunk. All of these postures are caused by abnormal muscle tone, also known as dystonia. Unlike the rhythmic movement related to dyskinesia, dystonia consists of sustained, deep muscular contractions which are often quite painful. Patients describe it as an uncontrollable cramping or tightening of their muscles.

Dystonia can occur as a symptom of the disease itself or as a side effect of levodopa therapy. Severe rigidity often manifests itself in abnormal postures, especially of the hands and feet, and can be alleviated by anti-Parkinson drugs. On the other hand, too much dopamine in the brain can cause dystonia by overstimulating muscular action.

Treatment: If you experience dystonias, keep track of when they occur. Is it before your medicine takes effect or after? If it's before Sinemet kicks in, your physician will probably either increase the amount of levodopa you take or have you take smaller doses more often. If your dystonia is a side effect of levodopa therapy, your doctor may reduce the amount of Sinemet you take, perhaps adding a dopamine agonist to make up the difference in anti-Parkinson effects.

Eating

Enjoying good food may become problematic for many parkinsonians, especially in the later stages of disease when chewing and swallowing are impaired. Even early on, a loss of appetite due to depression and/or lack of activity may disrupt normal eating patterns and even interfere with proper nutrition maintenance. (If you lack a healthy appetite, please see Chapter Five.) Other physical changes also may cause eating problems:

Handling Utensils

Patients with tremor and muscular rigidity may have trouble picking up food with forks and spoons; others are unable to grip the utensils. Embarrassing and frustrating, this incoordination may lead to a chronic appetite and weight loss.

Treatment: First of all, you should try to eat your biggest meals when you're most "on." Many people find they are hungriest and most able to eat at lunch; others find several smaller snacks, instead of three big meals, more appetizing and easier to manage.

A number of attractive and durable mealtime aids are available at medical supply stores and other outlets. They have been designed to enable you to eat with as much independence as possible, in spite of your motor limitations.

- Attachable plate guards and scoop dishes with contoured edges provide a rim on one side of the plate. Food, especially elusive vegetables such as peas and corn, can be pushed against the guard and thus onto a fork. These appliances also help prevent spills.
- Silverware with built-up plastic handles is more easily grasped. You can do it yourself with tubular foam padding purchased at your local hardware store.
- Soup spoons can be used instead of forks when eating small pieces of food.
- If your tremor affects your ability to hold a glass and sip from it, flexible plastic straws allow you to drink fluids with fewer spills. A lightweight mug, with a large handle for easy grasp, can be used if tremor is severe.
- Place rubber mats under plates, cups, and serving dishes to keep them from sliding.

Chewing

A parkinsonian's facial musculature may be affected by the disease, making the act of chewing difficult due to rigidity. Unfortunately, without the stimulation provided by vigorous chewing, your teeth are more susceptible to decay.

Treatment: If you have difficulty chewing because your teeth are loose or painful, make sure to visit a dentist. If you wear dentures, make sure they fit properly. Anti-Parkinson drugs will help your jaw muscles move more smoothly, making the act of chewing easier. A physical therapist will be able to suggest facial exercises that will help to strengthen chewing muscles.

Swallowing

The most common and problematic eating difficulty is dysphagia, a difficulty in swallowing. It usually occurs late in the disease.

Normally, swallowing begins when food is taken into the mouth then forced down the throat by the tongue. The presence of food in the throat starts the voluntary muscles of the upper esophagus contracting. These, in turn, start the involuntary muscles of the lower esophagus contracting, which pushes the food through the esophagus into the stomach.

In some patients, the swallowing difficulty arises from an inability to force the food down the throat and an inability of the voluntary muscles of the throat and esophagus to contract. This results in pooling of food in the throat. These patients complain of food getting stuck in their throat.

In very late stages of disease, patients who have difficulty swallowing may develop pneumonia. Normally, when food is in the throat, the throat closes off from the air passages that lead to the nose, as well as those that led to the lungs, thus preventing food from going into those areas. In some PD patients, however, pooling of the food in the throat may cause food to go into the lungs (aspiration), thereby resulting in cough or pneumonia.

Other swallowing difficulties may result from a failure of a valve that allows food to pass from the esophagus into the stomach. This may cause the patient to feel a bloated and burning sensation in the throat and chest. The burning sensation comes from the digestive juices of the stomach flowing into the esophagus via the faulty valve.

Treatment: To alleviate your food pooling in the back of your throat, take extra small bites of food, chew it thoroughly and swallow it carefully. Always completely swallow one morsel before putting more food into your mouth. Take your time; use an electric warming tray to keep your food hot so that you don't feel you have to rush. Remember to swallow excess saliva *before* you put food in your mouth.

Other tips for eating well and with pleasure:

- If you prefer using your own specially adapted utensils, bring them along when you go to restaurants. If you have trouble cutting your food at the table, ask the waitress to do it for you in the kitchen. Usually, they'll be happy to do it if asked in advance.
- Use a food processor to chop up good home-cooked meals so you can chew and swallow them easier, a healthier and more pleasurable alternative to baby foods.
- Use an insulated thermos with a push-button top that dispenses liquids easily. Fill it with a hot or cold beverage and keep it near you during the day.

Embarrassment

"My girlfriend, Rosemary, can't stand for anyone to see her tremor or walk with what she refers to as her 'Walter Brennan limp,' " admits Harry about the 33-year-old saleswoman you first met in Chapter Four. "It's barely noticeable. I see it only when I really look for it, but she's convinced everyone is staring at her. It's hard on me because I'd like to get out more."

Caspar, on the other hand, says he decided long ago not to feel embarrassed by his condition. "Almost right from the start, I had the bent posture, the slowness, and a pretty impressive tremor. At first, it bothered me some that people stared, but I never let it get in the way of my doing what I wanted. Most people don't mean any harm. I like the ones who come right out and ask what's wrong with me. The ones I could do without look away real quick like I have something contagious or disgusting."

Learning to handle the reactions of strangers to your condition may take some getting used to. You may resent their intrusion into what is a painful part of your personal life. As Caspar points out, however, most people are simply curious to know why you move so slowly, have tremors, or are dyskinetic. When you notice someone staring at you, you can respond in one of two ways: ignore them and continue with your activity, or take the time to explain to them that you have a neurological condition called Parkinson's disease that is causing you to move in abnormal ways. Some parkinsonians carry printed explanatory material from one of the national PD associations to give to people who express a sincere interest in the disorder. Whether you ignore or educate will depend both on your personality and on the time and energy you have available to speak at length to strangers.

If you decide to open the door of communication with someone curious about your condition, a little humor might make you both feel more comfortable. One woman tells people who inquire about her tremor that it's a new weight loss method designed to burn calories all day long, which always seems to get an empathetic laugh.

However you decide to approach the matter, you must not opt for the choice Rosemary made, which was to withdraw completely from society. First of all, it's likely that far fewer people than you think even notice you or your condition. Second, most people, as Caspar points out, mean no harm. Third, if you choose to withdraw for fear of being stared at, you risk developing far more serious problems than momentary embarrassment: loneliness and depression.

Employment

PD patients who are still working when they are diagnosed are usually anxious to keep their jobs and further their careers for both financial and personal reasons. For these people, the diagnosis of PD can be an especially devastating blow.

But PD does not necessarily mean an end to a full and productive work life. It may take a little reorganization or a shift from a high-stress job to another one that is less taxing, but with forethought and planning, you may be able to enjoy many more years of employment.

The first thing to do when considering your work situation is to take an honest look at your condition at this moment. Are you able to control your symptoms without many side effects on a regular basis? Do you have severe on-off periods? Is your balance affected or do you have gait problems that cause you to fall? How are your speech and communication skills? Are people able to understand you easily in conversation?

After you've made a realistic assessment of your stage of disease, make an appraisal of your job description and duties. Are you a manager or administrator, or does your job involve physical labor requiring muscle strength to lift and carry? Must you use fine motor skills to type or file? Are you on the phone a great deal or meeting with clients regularly?

Now match your own disabilities with your job requirements. Every patient will be different. Perhaps your balance and strength are good, but your fine motor skills are affected. If you work in a stockroom piling boxes, you'll be okay (as long as you remain aware of your capabilities). But if you're a word processor at a law firm with the same symptoms, you may have trouble doing your job.

Hugh, the 24-year-old marketing executive whom you met in Chapter One, has a job that utilizes his telephone communication skills a great deal. To maintain his position, he works very hard with a speech therapist to keep his voice strong and intelligible and knows that during his "off" periods he should busy himself with paperwork rather than try to speak with clients.

There may come a time when you are no longer able to perform certain aspects of your job responsibilities as they are set forth for you today. Does that mean you have to quit altogether? Maybe not. Consider making the following accommodative changes:

Modify Your Schedule: Many patients, in an effort to "make up" for their loss of function, actually try to *increase* their working hours and productivity. This creates a great deal of emotional and physical stress, which usually only exacerbate their symptoms and cause an even greater decline in output.

Instead, try to arrange a schedule that takes advantage of the times your body is working at its best. If you're most "on" in the morning, get to the office at 7:30 A.M. and leave at 3:30 P.M., before your worst "off" time kicks in. Or would coming in at 9:30 A.M., after rush-hour traffic, reduce your stress level? Would a long lunch hour give you time to stretch out somewhere and tackle afternoon chores with less "off" time? Many employers are willing to help you make adjustments, as long as you are able to perform the job assigned to you.

Learn to Adapt: Depending on your symptoms, you may need to find new ways to perform the duties expected of you. Many Parkinson's patients, for instance, suffer from micrographia, making their handwriting illegible. These employees should learn to use a typewriter or word processor (often much easier for a parkinsonian than writing by hand) to create memos or reports. If you have a secretary available to you, speak your correspondence into a Dictaphone and have her type it up. Some jobs, particularly those in sales and marketing, involve speaking on the telephone. If your speech is affected by your disease, you may need to adapt your telephone with an amplification device to increase the volume of your voice. (See Appendix I.)

If you are a manual laborer, your condition may affect your safety and the safety of others. Consider working with an occupational or physical therapist to modify the way you lift, carry, or otherwise use your body in your work. This will protect you from dangerous falls or secondary injuries such as muscle pulls or sprains. In addition, since you may not be objective about your abilities, confide in a co-worker about your condition so that he or she can monitor how you're performing your physical labor.

If you find yourself unable to perform the work you are assigned, check to see if the company will train you for another, less physically taxing job. State-funded rehabilitation projects may also be available if and when your condition prevents you from performing your job properly.

Choose Whom You Tell Carefully: If you're like most patients, you're afraid to tell your employer and/or colleagues about your condition. Know from the start that Parkinson's disease is considered a disability and you cannot be fired for simply having the disease. As long as you are able to perform the duties described in your job description, your boss cannot fire you because you are ill.

Unfortunately, some of your fears are indeed founded in reality. Especially in tough economic times when layoffs are common, Parkinson's disease patients have reason to fear that, if it came down to two equally qualified candidates, they may be the one to be dismissed. In addition, many firms have a tendency to offer "early retirement" to senior employees and to hire less costly junior replacements. A diagnosis of PD is sometimes the deciding factor in that instance as well.

Some of the same issues hold true for PD patients looking for a job as well. Should you tell a prospective employer about your illness? You are not required to by law, unless your condition would interfere with your job duties. And you cannot be denied the job solely on the basis of your disability. Nevertheless, many patients have found it very difficult to find employment with an obvious tremor or other noticeable symptom, even for a position they were perfectly capable of fulfilling.

While these situations are certainly reprehensible and in many cases illegal, it may be difficult—but not impossible—to challenge your superiors or potential employers. Consider seeing an attorney if you feel you've been unfairly dismissed or rejected.

But don't borrow trouble. You may be surprised at the amount of empathy and support you receive once you let your superiors and colleagues in on your condition. As mentioned in Chapter Six, your symptoms may have been evident to others long before you were diagnosed or even before you noticed them yourself. Tremor, loss of balance, and slowness in speech or movement also resemble a drinking or drug problem; many people may be relieved to hear you have a treatable, nonlife-threatening brain disorder.

Facial Masking

As you may remember from Chapter One, Beth's husband was the first to notice something amiss about his wife. He would catch her staring off into space often and not smiling as much as she used to. This lack of expression is known as having a *masked facies*, and it results from a combination of bradykinesia and rigidity affecting the facial musculature.

The muscles of the face control a number of different functions, including how often you blink your eyes and how well you chew your food. Human communication, too, depends to a large extent on the mobility of facial muscles. Expressions of sadness, hope, curiosity, and fear are made not only with words but with the movements of your mouth, eyes, and forehead. Keeping these muscles flexible and strong, then, will help you maintain essential communication skills.

Treatment: Anti-Parkinson drugs will alleviate most of the under-lying causes of facial masking. In addition, specific techniques have been developed to treat the results of PD not helped by drug therapy (see Eating and also Speech and Communication).

Gait Disturbances and Falling

Walking across the room, maneuvering through doorways and around furniture, reaching for a glass on a high shelf, leaning over to tie your shoes: These movements require literally thousands of electrical impulses traveling back and forth from the brain to the muscles. In a healthy brain, these movements take place semi-automatically, usually without the need for conscious direction.

As detailed in Chapter Two, the balance and coordination re-quired for safe movement are produced in the part of the brain called the striatum. The striatum sends messages concerning body position, posture, muscle coordination, and movement to other parts of the brain's motor control system with the aid of the neu-rotransmitter dopamine.

In a brain suffering from Parkinson's disease, however, this intricate system fails to work properly, resulting in several differ-ent kinds of movement disturbances. The most disabling of these is the inability of many PD patients to walk with an appropriate gait or maintain their balance. In general, the gait is more subdued, with the height of the steps lower and their length shorter. In addition to shuffling in this manner, many patients also lose the automatic swing of the arm opposite the moving leg.

Far more serious to the PD patient is a general loss of postural stability, otherwise known as balance. The healthy brain is able to automatically make the thousands of tiny body adjustments re-quired to keep us upright as we move forward or backward or when we bump against an object or pass through a doorway. For reasons not fully understood, this equilibrium is disturbed in Par-kinson's disease. Some PD patients, often in the later stages of disease but sometimes earlier, can be thrown off balance into a fall by just a slight push or simply by the anticipation of walking through a narrow doorway.

The gait disturbances PD causes often result in serious injuries and incapacity. Falls among PD patients are caused by a number of different, but interrelated, problems relating to proper movement. Some patients have difficulty walking properly from the very beginning of their disease, others not until much later. In addition, there are patients with severe balance problems who never experience festination or freezing and vice versa.

Listed below are some of the most common gait disturbances and ways to avoid falling because of them. For more general information about walking and exercise, see Chapter Five.

Festination: The typical forward posture of a PD patient promotes the tendency to walk quickly on the balls of the feet with the heels raised and the arms motionless. These shuffling steps often get shorter and faster with distance. When shuffling occurs:

- Stop walking.
- Make sure your feet are about 8 inches apart.
- Correct your posture by standing as straight as you can.
- Think about taking a large step.
- Imagine you are going to march or step over an object in your path.
- Lift your toes up first, then your knee, take the step, then place your heel down first.
- Roll onto the ball of your foot and toes.
- AT THE SAME TIME: Swing your opposite arm forward when taking a step. This improves the rhythm of walking and your appearance.
- Repeat this process with the other foot.

Propulsion and Retropulsion: If festination continues for more than a few steps, you may end up literally propelling yourself forward uncontrollably, a motion called propulsion. Eventually, you'll fall unless some object or person intervenes. Taking steps backward, after reaching for something high on a kitchen shelf, for instance, or backing out of in a closet, will result in a similar problem. This phenomenon is called retropulsion. Retropulsion also may result in dangerous falls.

Some patients find that the use of a cane will help stop the propulsion before a fall occurs. Retropulsion most often occurs when you are trying to reach for something higher than shoulder level. A good way to keep yourself from falling backward from this position is to first put one foot (preferably the one on your stronger side) about 8 to 12 inches behind you. This will give you leverage and support.

Freezing: Many parkinsonians suffer from the gait disturbance known as freezing. It is caused by a misfiring of the brain's neuroelectrical impulses. Freezing often occurs when a patient approaches narrow spaces such as doorways or between furniture, but sometimes it occurs for no apparent reason. When in a frozen position, patients are usually in a stooped posture with knees bent and heels off the ground, and the more they try to move, the more off-balance they become. Eventually, in frustration, they may try so hard to move that they fall instead.

If you are troubled by incidents of freezing, try the following:

- First, as soon as you freeze, stop trying to walk.
- If you're on your toes, place your heels on the floor.
- Straighten your knees, hips, and trunk, but DO NOT LEAN BACKWARD.
- Gently rock side to side, or have a caregiver stand in front of you, take your hands, and help gently rock you in the same way.
- Take some marching steps in place. Some patients find that having something to step over, like a piece of paper or a magazine, is helpful, too. Even simply *imagining* you have to step over something may help.
- Start taking a step forward by first lifting one knee up, taking the step, then placing your heel down first.
- Repeat with the opposite leg. Remember to keep your feet about 8 inches apart and to correct your posture if you feel you are beginning to lean forward or stoop.
- If you freeze at night when you walk to the bathroom or kitchen: make a path from your bed to the room using white socks on a carpet or white tape on a hard floor. As stated above, the action of stepping over something or lifting one foot high off the ground disengages the freezing.

Turning: When your balance is affected by the disease, turning around quickly will often cause you to fall. In addition, many patients tend to cross one foot in front of the other when turning, thereby tripping themselves. To make a safe turn, try thinking about making a U-turn, just as you would in an automobile: Never pivot on one foot by crossing your legs. Instead, walk in a forward direction into your turn. Walk around in a semicircle with your feet at least 8 inches apart.

Hallucinations

Small furry animals, groups of people having a party, long-deceased relatives sitting in your favorite chair, a strange feeling that someone is in the room with you when you are, in fact, alone. These are just a few of the hallucinations experienced by PD patients. About 25 percent of the parkinsonian population who have taken levodopa for more than three years or so are affected by hallucinations.

Almost all visions and delusions associated with PD drug therapy are benign. Nevertheless, most patients who experience hallucinations become quite frightened, not only by what they see but because they fear they are losing their minds. Hallucinations experienced by a PD patient are almost always related to drug therapy, not to progressive dementia. They can be quite disturbing, however, and you should speak with your physician or neurologist about them as soon as you experience them.

Treatment: Generally speaking, hallucinations occur during the later stages of disease, after the patient has been treated with levodopa therapy for three or more years. The patient may have become hypersensitive to levodopa or, rarely, to another anti-Parkinson drug. To lessen the frequency of hallucinations, your physician may reduce your Sinemet dosage, perhaps adding a dopamine agonist to make up the difference in effect. A number of adjustments and readjustments may have to be made before a satisfactory balance between symptoms and side effects is reached.

Hospitalization

It is particularly trying for the parkinsonian to be hospitalized. If at all possible, consult a neurologist before the patient is hospitalized, whether for a PD-related illness or otherwise. The neurologist may be able to tell you how the hospitalization will affect your parkinsonian symptoms. In addition, he may agree to consult with your surgeon or other members of the hospital staff to explain Parkinson-related needs and medication subtleties.

A patient admitted for a surgical procedure, for instance, is usually told not to "take anything by mouth" after 6:00 P.M. on the evening prior to surgery. This leaves the parkinsonian vulnerable to extreme rigidity and bradykinesia or severe tremors in the postoperative period, contributing to the trauma he may suffer and extending the convalescent period. In reality, most Parkinson medication could safely be taken with only a small sip of water right up to the time of surgery, and resumed shortly after the procedure if competent neurological advice was available to the surgery/anesthesia team.

Sometimes it's up to the patient and family themselves to educate the hospital staff about the intricacies of this complicated disease. It is, for instance, most helpful for medications to be left at the bedside if the patient is alert enough to deal with self-medication or an attentive spouse or caregiver is available to administer them on schedule. The typical hospital medication schedule of 9 A.M., 1 P.M., 5 P.M. and 9 P.M. may not fit the schedule of a particular parkinsonian's needs. Similarly, nursing personnel may not realize that small condiment or silverware packets on food trays or call lights located just out of reach amount to serious obstacles for parkinsonians with limited motor coordination.

The balance difficulties of many parkinsonians, combined with the restrictions of rails, tubes, and an unfamiliar environment, make independent mobility difficult even for the mild parkinsonian. The hospital staff should be made aware that although most parkinsonians do not appear frail or sick, they may need assistance in getting to the bathroom or elsewhere.

Exercise remains important to health maintenance, even within a hospital setting. Ask your physician what you might do to keep as mobile as possible. You may be able to do some exercises in bed or in a chair. With PD or not, people who remain sedentary for any length of time risk pneumonia, bed sores, phlebitis, contractures, and deconditioning.

All Parkinson patients and caregivers faced with hospitalization should be aware of the following "Patient's Bill of Rights," paraphrased from the formal American Hospital Association document:

1. The right to personal dignity, privacy, and courtesy
2. The right to know the identity of all physicians and other health-care providers who participate directly in your care
3. The right to receive full information about options for treatment
4. The right to confidentiality of your disclosures and medical records
5. The right to review your medical records

Most hospitals have an ombudsman or patient services representative to mediate difficulties for patients and families, and patients should not be shy about voicing concerns or problems—about medication, meals, and exercise, for instance—to such a person.

Kitchen Organization

If you spend a lot of time in the kitchen, consider reorganizing it to suit your special needs. Your goal is to make cooking and cleaning as easy as possible by limiting the amount of reaching and walking you have to do. Coffee and tea, for instance, should be stored as close as possible to the tea kettle; dishes and glasses stored over or beside the dishwasher or sink; pots and pans hung on the wall on hooks near the stove; bread stored near the toaster, etc. This way, even if you have impaired balance or slowness of movement, you can still enjoy your time in the kitchen without becoming overly taxed. Try preparing food—cutting vegetables, making sauces— while you remain seated at the kitchen table. Other hints for making your kitchen a safe and enjoyable haven include the following:

- Don't overestimate your fine motor skills when it comes to using a knife. If possible, let food processors do most of your cutting and chopping.
- If the handles on cabinets are too small to grab hold of, tie a long cloth around them so that you may grab the cloth and pull the cabinet open.
- Install roll-out shelves in lower cabinets to reduce the need to bend to reach things in back or having to first remove items in front to obtain items in back.
- Fill a lazy Susan with commonly used herbs and spices and set on the counter instead of in a cabinet.
- Use nonstick and lightweight pots and pans.
- Keep heavy kitchen items stored at shoulder or waist height so you don't have to strain to reach them.
- Cook as much food as you can during your "on" times. Divide portions into separate meals and freeze them.
- The use of a microwave oven eliminates the need for standing at the stove and stirring.
- Do not wax your kitchen floor; that will only make slipping and falling even easier.
- Use a cart with wheels to move items from room to room or from the kitchen to the table. You won't have anything to carry and you will have something to support you while you walk.
- Order Meals-on-Wheels from your local Council on the Aging if you live alone and cooking becomes too difficult for you to manage.

Medication Management

As a parkinsonian, you will take one or more medications to treat the symptoms of your disease several times a day, every day, probably for the rest of your life. Such a prognosis may seem daunting. Perhaps a daily vitamin or aspirin has been the extent of your drug use. And even if you're already on a daily medication regimen to treat high blood pressure, heart disease, or diabetes, the management of anti-Parkinson drugs may seem complicated to you at first.

As the doctor's partner in your treatment, however, it's up to you to learn as much as you can about the drugs you take and their effects on your own metabolism and body. Start by making a list of the medications prescribed to you. Look them up in Chapter Four and find out what symptoms they are best able to treat and what side effects they are likely to cause. Monitor how your body reacts as the therapy continues.

Many patients keep a daily diary of symptoms and side effects to help them evaluate the effects of the drugs on an hour-by-hour, day-to-day basis. Margaret, the schoolteacher whom you met in Chapter One, monitors her therapy carefully.

"Maybe it's from my experience as an educator, but I have a need to know exactly what's going on," Margaret admits. "I understand that there are ways to use the drugs so that they will work better for me and for a longer period of time. So about once or twice a week, I keep careful track of when I take my drugs, when my symptoms appear and disappear, and what side effects I have, if any." (See box below.)

As you may remember from Chapter Four, Margaret takes an extra pill on the days she substitute-teaches. "I learned two things by tracking my daily routine: First, most days I don't need a whole dose of medication before lunch. Why this is true I don't know. Most

---

Margaret's Daily Diary

8:00–9:00	Felt stiff when I woke up. Took first dosages (whole Sinemet, Parlodel) while still in bed. Waited ½ hour before they kicked in to get up.
9:00–12:30	Made myself breakfast. Played with my 4-year-old grandson in the yard. Did laundry. Did my daily exercises.
12:30–1:30	Started having trouble moving around at about 12:30. Asked my granddaughter to get my pill (½ dose of Sinemet and deprenyl) and took them about 15 minutes early. Unable to do much more than sit and watch the news on television for about 45 minutes.
1:30–4:00	Had lunch, then did a few errands. Started to slow down, got a little sleepy at about 2:30. Took a nap when I got home until I was ready for my next medication. (Took whole Sinemet, Parlodel.)

4:00–7:45	Once the meds kicked in (about 4:45), started dinner for family. About 5:30, started feeling very restless and edgy. Couldn't seem to sit still or calm down. That feeling wore off at about 6:00. Ate dinner early at about 6:30 so didn't take pill at 7:00 as usual (½ dose of Sinemet), but felt okay. Did dishes, talked with my daughter about problems my grandson is having in school. Felt stressed and could feel myself stiffening. Decided to take whole Sinemet (my "Cinderella" dose) at 7:45 so I could go to my PD support group meeting.
7:45–11:00	Once the Sinemet kicked in and I relaxed a little, I felt fine. Evenings and mornings seem best times for me. Went out for coffee (decaf!) with friends after meeting. Went to bed at 11:00, read for an hour, then fell easily to sleep.

Margaret tracked her reactions to her drug therapy every day for a week and noticed a number of patterns. She was stiff most every morning, took a real dip from midmorning to late afternoon, but then was dyskinetic (that restlessness and twitchiness) after her 4:00 dose.

With this information in her hand, she spoke to her doctor, who felt that she needed another medication adjustment. Her new drug schedule is:

8:00	one 10/100 Sinemet, Parlodel, deprenyl
11:00	one-half 10/100 Sinemet
12:00	lunch
1:30	one 10/100 Sinemet, Parlodel
4:00	one-half 10/100 Sinemet, deprenyl
6:00	dinner
7:00	one-half 10/100 Sinemet (or whole if going out)

of the people in my support group need most of their medication at the beginning of the afternoon. Second, when I'm under any kind of stress, like teaching, my symptoms worsen considerably and I need extra medicine to see me through. Trial and error, that's what my doctor told me PD therapy would be like. Boy, was he ever right!"

Try keeping a drug diary for a while to see if you can ascertain any pattern of disability that you and your doctor can help smooth out with medication adjustment. Less important in the early stages of disease, tracking daily fluctuations will become more essential the longer you take levodopa.

If you need assistance in organizing your medications and in remembering to take them, the following hints should help:

- If you take more than one medicine, keep a written schedule of when you should take each medicine. Use a different ink color to designate each medicine. Then you can see at a glance what drugs to take when.
- Purchase a sectioned container for a daily amount of pills. There are also pill boxes with alarms you can set to remind you to take your pills. Check with a medical supply company.
- Use a pill splitter to divide pills evenly. A straight-edged razor can also be used, with caution, as an alternative.
- Carry a flask of water for taking pills away from home.
- If you have trouble swallowing pills, drink some water first to moisten the throat or take them in Jell-O or applesauce.
- If you are severely disabled, make sure you keep a large-faced alarm clock, your medication and medication schedule, and a glass of water close to where you sit or lie during the day. Set the alarm to ring when medications are due. This will alleviate one need for constant caregiver attention.

Mood Swings

It is not uncommon for PD patients who are on medication to become moody and even uncharacteristically rude. The most obvious reason for such personality changes is the fact that the patient is suffering from an incurable, degenerative brain disease; that's often enough to make the best of us cranky and inconsolable.

On the other hand, mood fluctuations may be related to the amount and duration of drug therapy and can indicate potential levodopa overdose. In fact, some studies show that some patients experience mood fluctuations just before they start hallucinating or having delusions. That's why it's important for you to report any personality changes to your doctor immediately.

Treatment: Often, lowering the dosage of Sinemet and/or dopamine agonists will put the patient back on a more even emotional keel. Sometimes, simply getting more exercise and reviving old hobbies or finding new ones will help. If you find yourself emotionally overwrought, remember to consider the effects your moods have on your family and friends; thinking of others often has a therapeutic affect. If not, some patients—and their families—may want to consider seeing a psychologist or therapist for advice.

Nausea

Nausea, vomiting, and loss of appetite are common side effects of levodopa and/or dopamine agonist therapy. Most gastrointestinal discomfort associated with PD is caused by dopamine stimulation of the vomiting center in the brain, as described in Chapters Two and Four. Parkinson's disease itself may also cause nausea; because stomach muscles are affected by the disease, there is a delay in the emptying of the stomach. The PD patient may complain of feeling excessively full after even a small meal; this can also result in vomiting.

Treatment: Most of the drug-related side effects are short-lived and disappear as soon as your body adjusts to the medications. Some patients find that taking their medications with crackers and/or juice helps prevent an upset stomach. Unfortunately, some antivomiting, antinausea medications do more harm than good because they aggravate other PD symptoms. There are other drugs, however, that can help. See your physician if you are persistently plagued with nausea.

On-Off Effect

As described in depth in Chapter Four, levodopa becomes less effective the longer you take it. Although some patients take Sinemet for ten years or more with good results, most experience problems with the drug's effectiveness after five years. One result of this decline in levodopa's efficacy is called the "on-off effect." Instead of experiencing sustained relief from their symptoms, patients notice a marked drop in mobility and/or increase in tremor as one dose of medication wears off and before the next dose kicks in. (See Figure 3.)

As the drug continues to lose effectiveness and the disease process progresses in the brain, the "off" periods become longer and more pronounced. (See Caspar's case study at the end of Chapter Four.)

Treatment: The only way to reduce the on-off effect is to adjust your medication schedule and/or dosage. Some patients benefit from taking smaller doses of levodopa at shorter intervals. If your schedule calls for one 25/250 Sinemet at four-hour intervals from 7:00 A.M. to 7:00 P.M., for instance, your doctor may suggest half doses at two-hour intervals or a variation thereof. Or, as Caspar's doctor did, a dopamine agonist may be added to your drug regimen, helping to boost the original dose of Sinemet a bit. Dietary protein restriction (see Chapter Five) and/or the use of deprenyl

FIGURE 3.
THE ON-OFF EFFECT.
(FROM UNIVERSITY HOSPITAL, BOSTON DAY PROGRAM
FOR PARKINSON'S DISEASE PATIENTS.)

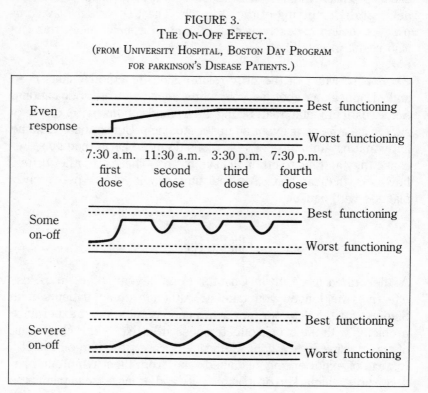

may also temporarily improve motor fluctuations. Your doctor may suggest you try the controlled-release form of Sinemet to see if it helps alleviate your on-off fluctuations. Unfortunately, as the disease progresses, the on-off effects will tend to get worse.

Parkinson's and Other Diseases

Other diseases may *coexist* with your Parkinson's disease. Indeed, patients with PD often suffer from other medical conditions, especially those associated with aging, such as heart disease and diabetes. Although the medication you take for PD should not, under most circumstances, interfere with your treatment for other conditions, and vice versa, there are some special considerations. If you see separate doctors—a neurologist for PD and a cardiologist for your heart condition—make sure that each of them is aware of *all* the drugs you take, as well as any other relevant medical information.

Glaucoma: Caused by abnormal pressure in the eye, glaucoma is a leading cause of blindness among the aging. This condition may be exacerbated by some of the anticholinergic drugs used to treat PD. If you have glaucoma, make sure your neurologist is aware of your condition so that he can prescribe anticholinergic therapy with caution. Patients with both conditions should be carefully monitored by an eye doctor.

Heart Disease: If you've had a recent heart attack or if your heart rhythm is irregular (arrhythmia), you may be especially sensitive to the side effects of some anti-Parkinson drugs. For some patients, even the slight drop in blood pressure caused by some of anti-Parkinson drugs may put them at risk for another heart attack. This does not mean you will be unable to take PD medication, but it will be up to you and your physician to decide if the drugs' benefits exceed their risk.

High Blood Pressure: In rare instances, certain drugs used to treat high blood pressure may worsen PD symptoms, namely those that block the action of the body's sympathetic nervous system. Clonidine (Catapres) is such a drug, and some patients are unable to take it without causing an increase in rigidity, bradykinesia, and/or tremor. There are many other antihypertension drugs that may work just as well to reduce your high blood pressure without exacerbating your PD. Make sure the doctor treating your high blood pressure is aware that you suffer from PD, and vice versa.

Another high-blood-pressure drug, though one rarely used, is methyldopa (Aldomet), and it also may be contraindicated in certain PD cases. Methyldopa is catabolized by the same enzyme that converts levodopa into dopamine, and it therefore competes with Sinemet in the body. This competition may decrease the beneficial effects of Sinemet. This does not occur in every patient, however. In fact, before Sinemet became available, methyldopa was combined with levodopa as a PD treatment. Nevertheless, both patient and physician should be aware of the potential interaction between the drugs.

Diuretics (water pills) are frequently used to treat patients with high blood pressure or heart disease. Water pills produce a decrease in the amount of body fluid, which may result in dizziness on standing (orthostatic hypertension). This dizziness is more likely to affect PD patients, particularly those who take Sinemet or a dopamine agonist.

Stomach and Intestinal Diseases: There have been isolated reports relating bleeding ulcers to Sinemet and the dopamine agonists, although no direct cause-and-effect relationship has been established.

As discussed under "Swallowing" (see Eating), the valve between the esophagus and the stomach may open at the wrong time, resulting in gastric juice flowing back into the esophagus, which causes an inflammation. This may be followed by nausea and vomiting, which will result in further inflammation. Patients who have a hiatus hernia are especially vulnerable to this complication. This inflammation may result in erosion of the wall of the esophagus, which can lead to bleeding.

Patients who have a hiatus hernia and who take anti-Parkinson drugs should follow an appropriate diet prescribed by their physician. In addition, such patients may require antacids or other measures to decrease the inflammation. Patients with a history of liver disease, jaundice, or hepatitis should have liver function tests before taking anti-Parkinson drugs. These tests may have to be repeated periodically.

Orthopedic Conditions: At any stage of disease but especially when loss of balance is involved, PD patients may fall and break a bone. Those patients with severe tremors or severe dyskinesia will require specific medication adjustment to lessen these symptoms so that the broken bone can be set.

Cancer: In general, the influence of a cancer on PD is unknown. There have been a few reports in which the use of levodopa has been associated with the growth of melanoma (a tumor that arises from cells in the skin that produce the pigment melanin), a kind of skin cancer, but there is no evidence of a direct cause and effect relationship. Again, balancing benefits and risks is the duty of both you and your physician.

Posture Correction

As a result of immobility and the disease itself, many Parkinson's disease patients develop a stooped posture. Rigidity, as you may remember, is another term for the abnormal muscle tone or state of contraction caused by the lack of dopamine in the striatum. When the muscles in your neck, back, shoulders, hips, and knees are affected, you are forced to bend forward. Not only is this posture uncomfortable and unattractive, but it contributes to the breathing problems, dystonias, and gait disturbances associated with Parkinson's disease.

Treatment: Although anti-Parkinson drugs will help improve and maintain your posture, a full program of physical therapy, including, but not limited to, those exercises illustrated in Chapter Five, should be instituted as soon as you notice any postural changes.

Restlessness

Patients occasionally experience extreme restlessness. You may feel as if you simply cannot sit still. You may pace or fidget uncontrollably. The medical term for this is akathisia, and it is often caused by anti-Parkinson drugs.

Treatment: In most cases, akathisia is intermittent and patients prefer to simply live with their restlessness. If it is troublesome enough, your physician may suggest a reduction in Sinemet.

Sexual Dysfunction

Many Parkinson's disease patients experience sexual problems, including loss of libido and difficulties in performing the sexual act. Some of these problems are related to the disease, others are due to normal aging, and still others are a combination of many different factors. Indeed, human sexuality involves every aspect of the nervous system, from the simplest nerve transmission to the most complex cognitive function. As advanced as neurology has become, it cannot fully explain how the mechanisms of attraction, arousal, stimulation, and orgasm work in each individual.

As we age, both our physical bodies and our emotional makeup undergo a series of changes that often dramatically affect our sexual lives. Add a chronic illness like Parkinson's disease, and sex is often the last thing on a long list of priorities. However, although other aspects of PD may seem more important to you than sex, intimate behavior is a natural, integral part of all our lives. For your sake, and for your partner's sake, don't ignore it.

As you know, most Parkinson's disease patients are in their 60s and 70s. By this time, both women and men have experienced physical changes that involve their sexual habits. Once a woman enters menopause, for instance, hormonal changes often lessen the production of vaginal lubrication, making sexual relations uncomfortable or painful. In addition, with less estrogen, the vaginal wall becomes thinner, and intercourse may feel rough or scratchy. Older men may find that it takes longer to achieve an erection and that the erection is not as firm as it once was. A decrease in the amount of ejaculate and decreased force of ejaculation also may result from the aging process. This may lead to feelings of inadequacy and a decline in libido.

At any age, sexual ability and desire may be affected by a number of physical factors, medication (of any kind) and stress being the most prevalent. Parkinson's disease itself adds several other complications. For one thing, many scientists believe that dopamine is directly involved in the sexual response. This may explain why some PD patients experience a loss of libido. Rigidity and bradykinesia may inhibit the mechanical aspects of lovemaking. For example, slowness in turning over in bed may make it difficult for an affected male partner to assume the missionary position; rigidity in a woman may not allow her to open or raise her legs as she once did in the same position.

Many commonly used drugs, especially antidepressant drugs and anticholinergic PD therapy, may impair sexual function, usually by resulting in delayed ejaculation and impairment of penile erection. How anti-Parkinson medications affect sexual behavior in women has not yet been studied.

So far, we've talked only about the physical aspects of sexuality and Parkinson's disease, but more than likely, your self-esteem took a blow from the diagnosis of PD. You may feel less attractive and/or "less of a man or woman." You may feel afraid of being unable to perform or enjoy sexual relations as much as before you had Parkinson's. You may even be afraid that your partner is staying with you out of pity and could never really be sexually attracted to you again.

Guilt is perhaps the biggest sexual turnoff in the world, and both you and your partner may well have built a wall of guilt between you. You feel guilty because you've become a burden or because you feel you're no longer attractive. Your partner feels guilty because he or she feels just a bit resentful of your disease.

Finally, if your sexual partner is also your primary caregiver, you may have difficulty in discarding your "role" as a patient for the equality good sexual relations require. If your partner must cut your meat for you because you lack fine motor skills, or should he or she have to clean up after your occasional incontinence, then seeing yourself or your partner as sexually desirable can be quite difficult.

Treatment: There is no one solution to sexual dysfunction experienced by Parkinson's disease patients. The purely physical problems are, in many instances, the most easily solved. Vaginal dryness can be alleviated by the use of water-soluble lubricating jellies such as K-Y jelly. Anti-Parkinson drug therapy will alleviate some of the stiffness and rigidity that may interfere with finding a satisfying position for sexual intercourse or manual stimulation.

Honesty, understanding, and planning between you and your partner are the keys to resuming and maintaining a healthy and satisfying sex life. You might think that discussing and planning sexual activity will take the "thrill" of it away. In fact, anticipation and planning can add both excitement and self-confidence to your lovemaking.

Perhaps the most crucial element in the parkinsonian's sexual life is timing. Plan to have sexual relations when your medications are working best. Many parkinsonians function best in the morning or early afternoon. Choosing a time that works for both you and your partner also allows you to emerge from your roles as caregiver and patient. For that hour or two, force yourself to leave your other, disabled self behind and your partner to cast aside any nursing notions. Instead, become equals in the quest for mutual pleasure.

Be as direct as you can about your sexual needs and preferences and encourage your partner to do the same. If you feel awkward and clumsy performing sexual intercourse the way you always have in the past, ask your partner to try some new positions with you. If actual penetration is difficult or impossible, look for other alternatives to satisfaction. Mutual masturbation or artificial stimulation (dildos and vibrators) are options that should be considered without hesitation if both of you feel comfortable about them. Consider seeking the advice of a therapist if you are unable to break down some of the barriers to communication.

Most important, both you and your partner should know that you can still touch and embrace without having it necessarily lead to sexual intercourse. The sexual act is just one part, albeit an important one, of a loving relationship. Enjoy the pleasure that comes from gentle caresses, hugs, and kisses.

Shopping

Lifting and reaching at the grocery, trying on clothes at department stores, lugging packages to the car, and waiting in line, any or all of these tasks can make shopping a nightmare for a PD patient.

Luckily, there are a number of solutions to your shopping problems. First of all, one of the few real benefits of having a chronic illness is that it entitles you to park in the precious few handicapped parking spaces located near most major shopping areas. (Check with your city hall or Department of Motor Vehicles to get a special license plate.) That will alleviate some of the stress involved in finding a parking place and the physical strain of having to walk long distances.

If you are retired or work only part-time, you can shop during off-hours when stores are less crowded. To shop for groceries, first make a list of what you need and organize it by the aisles in which the items are found. Some stores even offer personal helpers to push your cart and reach for items. If your local grocery doesn't have this service, bring or request wooden pickup tongs to help you reach for high items. Consider using grocery stores that deliver. That way, you can simply call in your order and wait.

Buying clothes may also be difficult for you, especially if your symptoms prevent you from trying them on with ease. Some patients have better luck—and more fun—going with a friend who can help them dress and undress. Another option is to buy clothes off the rack and bring them home without trying them on. As long as you can return them, then you can try them on at your leisure. If you're not on a tight budget, hire a personal shopper to do all the legwork for you. Other hints for painless shopping:

- Use drive-up facilities available at banks, fast-food restaurants, and some convenience stores.
- Call stores before you go to make sure they have the items you need.
- Shop from mail-order catalogs.

Shortness of Breath

"I can never seem to catch my breath anymore," Beth complains. "You'd think I had run the marathon the way I gasp, even though

I've only walked from the kitchen with a cup of tea." Indeed, many PD patients complain of a tightness in their chest that prevents them from taking in sufficient oxygen.

This may be due to rigidity and bradykinesia of the chest wall muscles which prevent the lungs from expanding. Work with a speech or physical therapist on deep breathing exercises (or try the one described under Stress). Please note that some cases of breathlessness could be caused by heart or lung disease, therefore inform your doctor if it persists or is painful.

Skin Care

Good skin care is often a neglected area of health maintenance in the PD patient, mainly because it presents a confusing picture. On the one hand, seborrheic dermatitis (dandruff) and oil/waxy skin around the face and neck resulting from overactive sebaceous glands are frequently characteristics of Parkinson's disease. On the other hand, like most older adults, parkinsonians may discover that skin over most of the body is excessively dry, especially in cold weather.

Treatment: Mineral oil (available scented as baby oil) or heavier lubricant creams such as Nivea applied immediately after bathing are excellent means of retaining moisture in the skin. A mild astringent such as witch hazel can be used to reduce surface oiliness. A variety of over-the-counter antidandruff shampoos are also available. Salicylic acid formulations are more effective than the less expensive zinc oxide shampoos, and lack the unpleasant odor typical of coal tar preparations.

Inexpensive quality skin-care products and makeup suited to dry or sensitive skin are available in drugstores. The key moisturizing ingredient in most luxury facial creams is imidazolidinyl urea. Check labels on medications and cosmetics just as you do at the grocery store.

(Please note: Beware of bath oils and similar products added to the bath water; falls in slippery tubs can be hazardous.)

Sleep Disorders

Insomnia and/or impaired sleep will decrease the daytime function of the PD patient. As we get older, our sleep patterns change. Many of us have more trouble getting and staying asleep as we age. In addition, the symptoms of PD may contribute to sleep problems. Tremor, for instance, may occur almost anytime during the night, but most especially during the early stages of sleep. Stiffness may affect your ability to get comfortable and stay relaxed enough to sleep. About one-third of all patients also experience periodic leg movements—jerking back and forth—which can awaken them, even from a sound sleep.

Anti-Parkinson medications also have the potential to disturb your ability to sleep. Levodopa therapy increases the activity of three neurotransmitters: dopamine, serotonin, and norepinephrine, all of which are involved in the process of sleep. For some patients, levodopa causes vivid dreams and nightmares, which may first keep them from falling asleep for fear of dreaming and then wake them up in fright.

Sleep apnea, an abnormal breathing pattern, may be related, in a few rare instances, to sleep problems in a PD patient. It occurs when muscles in your esophagus overrelax during sleep, thereby causing an obstruction of normal airflow. Unable to breathe for a moment, you wake up gasping.

Treatment: Finding a balance between relief of PD symptoms and avoidance of side effects is especially important to sleep management. For the most part, you shouldn't take a dose of Sinemet or an anticholinergic close to your bedtime for two reasons: First, anti-Parkinson medications tend to accumulate in most patients; it's likely that you already have enough in your system to last through the night, and any more might cause nightmares or difficulty in falling asleep. Second, you must always keep the long-term effects of drug treatment in mind: the less medication you take on a daily basis, the longer the anti-Parkinson effects will last and with fewer side effects. Many patients would rather not "waste" a dose of Sinemet on hours when they need it least.

On the other hand, some patients (Hugh, for example) may

choose to take a small dose of levodopa before they go to bed so that they can both move better during the night and get up more easily in the morning. Depending on their total daily dosage, that may be, for them, a perfectly acceptable trade-off.

Apart from medication adjustment, most patients simply need to develop better sleep habits. Many patients who complain of insomnia also report taking several long naps during the day. Staying active instead of resting will help ensure you're tired enough to sleep well at night. If you need rest, try a passive activity such as watching television or flipping through a magazine. Most important of all, do not sleep simply because you're bored. Find new hobbies and activities to fill your time. This will help you avoid depression and loneliness as well.

Other tips for better sleep management include the following:

- Exercise regularly.
- Modify your definition of "normal" sleep requirements. As we age, we generally require less sleep. If you feel refreshed after just four, five, or six hours of sleep, don't try for more. Instead, stay up an extra couple of hours so that you'll wake up at 6:00 or 7:00 A.M. having had just enough sleep.
- If you do wake up in the middle of the night, don't try to force yourself back to sleep. Read or watch television quietly until you feel drowsy again.
- Some patients find that establishing a ritual to follow helps prepare their bodies and minds for sleep. A routine of taking a warm bath, having a cup of tea, and/or reading for an hour after getting into bed may make falling asleep easier to do.
- If you and your doctor decide that a levodopa overdose is causing your nighttime problems, you may want to consider having a small protein snack such as a piece of cheese or glass of milk before bed. Conversely, if you wake up severely rigid or tremorous, you may need to take a dose of Sinemet. Again, discuss the matter with your physician.

Speech and Communication

Losing the ability to communicate with the people around you can be one of the most isolating aspects of Parkinson's disease. About one-half of all individuals with PD develop difficulty with their speech. Other individuals, even after years with Parkinson's disease, experience little or no change in their speech.

The speech changes that may occur are related to incoordination and reduced movement of muscles that control respiration (breathing), phonation (voice), articulation (pronunciation), prosody (rhythm, intonation, rate of speaking), and facial expressions. You may find that you have some or all of the following symptoms:

- *Soft voice volume:* This is often the first change in speaking ability that is noted. As time goes on, voice volume may be severely reduced to the point of inaudibility.
- *Fading voice:* At the beginning of a sentence, your voice is strong, but fades as you continue to talk.
- *Monotone voice:* The voice stays at the same level, lacking variation and expression.
- *Changes in voice quality:* The voice sounds breathy, tremulous, or high-pitched, or perhaps hoarse and strident.
- *Unwanted hesitation before speaking:* You may have difficulty initiating speech and getting a steady voice from the beginning of a conversation or even from the beginning of each sentence.
- *Indistinct pronunciation:* Words are slurred and word endings are omitted: final consonant sounds (for example, the "k" in book, the "l" in bell) are not clear.
- *Fast rate of speaking:* Syllables and words are crowded and run together without the usual pauses. There may also be a progressive acceleration of words toward the end of a sentence.
- *Uncontrollable repetitions:* Words, phrases, or sentences are repeated unintentionally and uncontrollably.
- *Lack of facial expression:* You may find that your face is less mobile and expressive and that smiling, frowning, grinning, and other facial movements are difficult.

Treatment: It is strongly advised that a certified speech-language pathologist evaluate your particular speech difficulties. The speech-language pathologist can provide a treatment program and make recommendations specific to your individual needs, as well as provide helpful information for your family. In the meantime, here are a few general suggestions for improving your speech:

- Keep in mind that your ability to speak clearly now requires your conscious and deliberate effort and attention.
- Take a breath before you start to speak and pause between every few words or even between each word.
- If low volume is a problem for you, think of shouting your words.
- Exaggerate your pronunciation of words. Force your tongue, lips, and jaw to work hard as you speak. Enunciate as if your listener is hard of hearing and needs to read your lips.
- Finish saying the final consonant of a word before starting to say the next word. Precise word endings are necessary to differentiate word meanings: for instance, the difference between "bag" and "bat." You should develop an awareness of the feel of your lips and tongue as they form each sound.
- Express your ideas in short, concise phrases or sentences. Long, involved sentences are often impossible for your listener to comprehend.
- To help you vary your facial expression, make your self conscious of how facial changes look and feel. Make faces at yourself in a mirror: smile, frown, laugh, grin, pout, whistle, and puff out your cheeks.
- Exaggerate facial motions as you recite the alphabet, count numbers, or read a poem or newspaper article.
- Face your listener. It will be easier for both of you to communicate if you have each other's full attention.
- Encourage your family and friends to ask you to speak louder or repeat yourself.
- Most important of all, speak for yourself. Don't get into the habit of letting others do your talking for you.
- If you live alone or spend a great deal of time by yourself, read a newspaper article into a tape recorder every day, and then play back the tape to see if you notice any change in your speech such as slurring or loss of amplification. Then practice words and phrases that give you.
- In those cases where speech is severely impaired, supplement your speech by writing. In addition, there are a number of aids and devices, such as printed charts, which allow patients to point to letters, words, or pictures to communicate. If your main problem is a weak voice, the use of an amplification

device may help to improve your voice volume so that you can be more readily understood. However, if you also suffer with slurred speech, uneven rate, and lack of voice variation, it is unlikely that amplification can be of much benefit. It may even exaggerate the overall problem.

(For more information about amplification devices and other communication aids, see Appendix I.)

Stress

There is little doubt that our psychological state has an effect on our physical body. Although a clear physiological relationship has yet to be defined, many physicians believe that stress may exacerbate a number of medical conditions, including high blood pressure, heart disease, and even cancer. Many parkinsonians report that their symptoms, especially tremor, get worse when they are under physical or emotional stress.

Stress is associated with the "fight-or-flight response," which occurs automatically in reaction to perceived danger. The perception of danger prompts a series of reactions in the body, ending with the release of several hormones including epinephrine and norepinephrine, which are also two powerful neurotransmitters. These chemicals prepare the body to quite literally either run or fight by causing the pulse to quicken, muscles to tense, blood pressure to rise, and the senses to sharpen.

Being alert can be very helpful, but if the body is constantly trying to perform its complicated functions under these heightened conditions, damaging side effects are sure to result. The hormone cortisol released under stress, for instance, is linked to a rise in blood cholesterol levels, a key risk factor for atherosclerosis and heart disease.

The connection between stress and PD is even more direct. When your body reacts to stress, brain chemistry is dramatically altered. Not only is more norepinephrine produced, but more acetylcholine is produced as well, creating a larger imbalance between these chemicals and the PD brain's depleted stores of dopamine. As discussed in Chapters Two and Four, this imbalance is directly linked to the resting tremor and rigidity of Parkinson's disease. That is why anticholinergics, drugs that work to inhibit the action of acetylcholine, successfully treat PD symptoms. In addition, the muscular tension that accompanies the fight-or-flight response only adds to the rigidity and bradykinesia experienced by most PD patients.

Understanding the physiological reasons why stress causes your tremor to emerge, however, does not necessarily help you or the medical profession solve the problem. One challenge is that, except for extreme situations, such as a divorce or the death of a loved one, a clear definition of stress itself is unavailable. One man's relaxing day at the beach could be sheer torture for someone whose idea of fun is a day of making business deals at the office. Also, many of us define stress far too narrowly. Stress is physical as well as emotional—your body experiences stress every time you shovel snow or carry a bag of groceries up a flight of stairs. For someone suffering from a disease like Parkinson's, physical stress is often directly related to an increase in symptoms. But stress can be positive as well as negative. The emotions attached to the birth of a child may create as much stress as the death of a spouse.

Not everyone responds to stress in the same way; some people overtly panic over the slightest mishap while others never blink an eye when disaster occurs. But it could be that the outwardly calm person is seething inside, causing his body chemistry to produce more acetylcholine and norepinephrine over a longer period of time. The person who expresses anger, frustration, and panic in a more open way may be able to calm down, and therefore regain the body and brain's equilibrium, far more quickly.

Treatment: Needless to say, stress and how it affects a PD patient is yet another completely individual aspect of the disease. So, too, is the treatment of it. The first step is for you to evaluate how much emotional and physical stress you have in your life. Are you worried about your marriage? Is your job a stressful one? Have you come to terms, at least for the time being, with your PD? Do you get terribly nervous and upset when you meet new people?

Once you've located the stressful areas in your life, see if there are ways to resolve them. Set realistic goals for attacking these obviously large and complicated problems. See a marriage counselor or therapist once a week. Arrange a vacation from work or rearrange your work schedule so that you have more free time.

Now for the hard part: You must learn to relax. Yes, there is an art to relaxing, and like any art, it takes practice and concentration to achieve it. In fact, for many people, *trying* to relax can be a stressful activity in itself. Nevertheless, managing stress is an integral part of overall therapy for Parkinson's disease and it's up to you to choose a "relaxation plan" that works for you. Among the options:

Exercise: Physical activity is a great way to relieve tension. Once again, brain chemistry is involved, this time in a positive way. Studies show that during exercise tranquilizing chemicals called endorphins are released in the brain causing your body to relax quite naturally. Stretching and strengthening the muscles affected by PD are added benefits.

Deep Breathing: Proper breathing is one of the most effective techniques for reducing stress. As mentioned in the Speech and Communication section, however, many parkinsonians do not breathe properly because of rigidity of the chest and abdominal muscles. Nevertheless, you should attempt this breathing exercise whenever possible:

1. Stop whatever task is making you feel stressed.
2. Relax your shoulders and arms.
3. Slowly exhale through your nose.
4. Now take a deep breath, letting your abdomen and then your chest fill with air.
5. Exhale slowly and repeat until your breathing is regular and steady. As you do, concentrate on each breath.
6. Feel relaxed and in control.

Develop a Hobby: Doing something you really enjoy and doing it every day can help you reduce stress. Gardening, cooking, and participating in a club or organization are just a few of the many options available.

Meditate: The relaxation response, developed by Boston physician Herbert Benson in the 1970s, relies on the tradition of transcendental meditation to evoke a calm, relaxed attitude in patients under stress. Many books are available on this and other meditation techniques.

No matter what approach you take to reducing stress in your life, if you're successful you're likely to see some reduction in your PD symptoms. Eating the right kinds of food, getting enough sleep, and talking with friends or a therapist about the problems you face will also help you prevent stress from becoming a negative force in your life.

Sweating

Another unusual nonmotor symptom in PD is episodes of excessive sweating not triggered by any change in temperature. These episodes of sweating can actually soak the patient's clothes. It appears that PD may involve a loss of control of the sweat glands in some patients. They then respond to normal stimuli—stress, a slight rise in temperature—with excessive sweating.

Treatment: Some anti-Parkinson drugs, in particular the anticholinergics, may help reduce excessive sweating. Levodopa, however, may cause sweating.

Swelling of the Feet

Swelling of the feet probably results from the inability of the rigid leg muscles to massage fluid from the feet back to the heart. Such fluid normally accumulates in the feet through the effects of gravity. Rarely, drugs such as Symmetrel and some of the dopamine agonists may result in swelling of the feet.

Treatment: Simply elevating your feet onto a stool or ottoman usually alleviates swelling, as does wearing support hose during the day. However, if the condition becomes pronounced, talk to your physician about it. Such swelling may be unrelated to PD but instead indicate heart or vessel disease. If the swelling is PD-related, your doctor may decide to adjust your medications or, rarely, to prescribe water pills to reduce the fluid in your body.

Transfers

Patients often have trouble standing after sitting on a low surface, such as a chair, car seat, or bed. To stand, always bring your buttocks close to the edge of the chair. Keep your feet at least eight inches apart, with one slightly in front of the other. Use momentum by rocking your trunk quickly back and forth three times. On the third time, bring your shoulders forward, just past your knees, push down on your hands, and straighten up.

Chairs and sofas that are soft and low are hard to rise from without help. A straight-back chair with a firm seat and arms helps in both sitting and rising. A firm cushion or chair risers can be used to make chairs the correct height. The seat should never be lower than knee height. Chairs that automatically raise and tilt the seat forward are available and helpful.

Tremors

Tremor is the most obvious symptom of Parkinson's disease, affecting about 75 percent of all patients. Tremor generally occurs early in the course of disease, but may never occur in some patients. The most common tremor occurs when the muscles are at rest, with a frequency of about 4–5 cycles a second. The tremor can be a to-and-fro motion of a limb, or it can be associated with more complex thumb and digit movements commonly referred to as the "pill-rolling" effect.

Most tremors are variable and intermittent, usually disappearing during sleep and increasing under stress. They may start in one arm or leg, then move to the other side, or just involve one limb all the time. They can involve all limbs as well as the jaw and lower facial muscles, even the lips.

What causes tremor in PD is unknown. The variability of tremor reflects its complex linkage with neuronal circuits everywhere, as evidenced by its fluctuating severity in response to mood, motor activity, general health, posture, and even time of day.

Treatment: All anti-Parkinson drugs relieve tremor to some degree, occasionally reducing it completely. Parkinsonian tremor is a resting tremor, which means it is most evident when the affected limb is still. If you suffer from tremor, you may have noticed that your hand, arm, or leg is free of tremor when you are working the muscles of that limb. Sometimes a slight movement or change of posture may arrest the tremor for a while, although it is likely to reappear within a few moments. In addition, some patients are able to stop a tremor just by concentrating on it.

Like most other manifestations of PD, tremor tends to be aggravated by stress or anxiety. Unfortunately, if you're nervous *and* trying to stop the tremor, you'll most likely only make it worse. Instead, take a few long, deep breaths and try to relax. Playing with a paper clip or other small object may also help under these circumstances. For more information, read the Stress entry above.

Urinary Problems

Both Parkinson's disease and the drugs used to treat it may cause urinary tract difficulties in some patients. They consist of urgency (a strong desire to void), frequency, hesitancy in starting to void, difficulty in completing voiding, and incomplete voiding with dribbling.

Rarely, a patient may be unable to void. Likewise rarely, incontinence affects PD patients in the late stages of disease when control of the muscles of the bladder and bowel have been completely lost. Accidental incontinence may occur earlier, however, if the bradykinetic patient cannot get to the bathroom in time.

PD results in voiding difficulties because the muscles in the bladder become rigid and bradykinetic, thus decreasing the ability of the bladder to contract and expel urine. In addition, some anti-Parkinson drugs, especially the anticholinergics and amantadine may increase these symptoms.

Treatment: Medication adjustment may alleviate most urinary problems: a slight increase in Sinemet and or a decrease in anticholinergics may be in order if your problems are persistent. Some patients feel more comfortable wearing absorbent undergarments to avoid embarrassing situations.

Parkinson's disease does not usually cause serious urinary tract disorders. If you are experiencing pain, burning, or markedly different urinary habits, see your doctor. In men, this difficulty may suggest problems with the prostate gland. Women may suffer from a laxness of the vagina or uterus, with secondary pressure on the bladder. Diabetes and urinary tract infections may also cause irritation of the bladder, resulting in voiding problems.

Vision Problems

The sense of sight is controlled by tiny muscles and nerves, some of which may be affected by both PD and drug therapy. Parkinson's disease itself does not cause loss of vision or blindness. If there are marked difficulties with eye movement, a diagnosis other than, or in addition to, PD should be considered.

Patients with PD report difficulty reading, blurred vision when looking closely at objects, and occasionally double vision. A decrease in night vision also occurs in some cases. In many PD patients, the eyes move with a kind of cogwheeling rigidity similar to the abnormal tone that is felt in the muscles of the limbs of patients with PD. The patient has to work hard to make out the sequence of letters and words and moving down the page to the next line. The problem is impaired coordination of the muscles that move the eye. The eyes also freeze, festinate, and travel slowly across the printed page.

In addition to being affected by the disease itself, your vision may be disturbed by some of the anti-Parkinson medications you're taking, including the anticholinergics. They will cause the pupils to widen slightly, resulting in blurry vision. Double vision may result when the muscles don't control the eyes well enough and they look at two different points in space.

Parkinson's disease patients may also develop bloodshot, irritated eyes which feel crusty and which may burn and itch, commonly known as conjunctivitis. This occurs because the normal blinking-wetting activity of the eyelids diminishes.

Treatment: Vision problems caused by PD are usually alleviated with Sinemet therapy; otherwise a reduction of anticholinergics may be in order. If you suffer from conjunctivitis, have your physician recommend a brand of artificial tears or another wetting solution available at your pharmacy. If your vision problems make reading difficult, you might consider listening to books on cassettes available at most libraries and bookstores.

Writing

Do the letters in your handwriting become smaller and blurrier the longer you write? If so, you are one of many PD patients suffering from micrographia, or the tendency to write small. Your fine motor skills are being affected by the lack of dopamine in the brain, causing your hand to make smaller and smaller movements. In addition, if you look carefully, you may see that the lines of the letters are also squiggly, indicating a tremor imposed upon the rigidity.

Treatment: Anti-Parkinson drugs should correct most of your writing difficulties, especially in the early stages of disease. For patients who continue to have trouble writing, try using a pen or pencil with an extra large body. Stop writing and pick up your arm frequently, at least once or twice a sentence. Many patients find that writing with a felt-tip pen is easiest.

Zest and Zeal

The power of positive thinking should never be underestimated. No one can say for certain how much of our general health is due to our state of mind. The same is true for the way we cope with chronic illness. If you wake up looking forward to the day's events and activities—even the challenges—with hope and confidence, it's almost certain you'll feel in better control of your symptoms than if you face the day with depression and despair. Never forget, too, the power of a great big belly laugh. As hard as it may seem at times, try to find some humor in your own situation and look for the funny, wonderful things in the world around you. Indeed, laughter is the best medicine in the world.

How Much Do You Know About Parkinson's Disease?

1) A medication commonly used to treat tremor in Parkinson's disease is:
   a) Artane
   b) Vitamin E
   c) Vitamin C
   d) Xanax

2) The chemical in the brain which is primarily depleted or decreased in Parkinson's disease is:
   a) Dopamine
   b) Acetylcholine
   c) Serotonin
   d) Bradykinin

3) Sinemet contains two ingredients, levodopa and:
   a) Kemadrin
   b) Parlodel
   c) Carbidopa
   d) Vitamin B_6

4) Which of the following is *not* a cardinal symptom of Parkinson's disease?
   a) Slow movements
   b) Rigid muscles
   c) Tremor
   d) Depression

5) Symptoms of overmedication include all of the following *except:*
   a) Abnormal involuntary movements
   b) Sleep disturbances
   c) Mental changes
   d) Rigidity

6) Which one of the following is *not* a safety precaution to keep in mind when one experiences walking difficulties?
   a) Keeping feet wider apart when walking
   b) Wearing sneakers
   c) Using your hands to touch furniture and railings
   d) Making U-turns
   e) Remembering to stand up straight

7) If a person is experiencing some difficulty moving in the middle of the morning, the *first* thing to do is:
   a) Call the doctor
   b) Take an extra dose of Sinemet

   c) Cancel plans for walking in the afternoon

   d) Note the time of day, when the last Sinemet was taken, and see if the problem occurs tomorrow

8) Of the following activities, which is *not* recommended for most patients?

   a) Swimming

   b) Gardening

   c) Roller skating

   d) Stretching and range-of-motion activities

9) Sinemet works most effectively if taken:

   a) Half an hour before meals with water or juice

   b) Half an hour after meals with water or juice

   c) Just before eating breakfast, lunch, or dinner

   d) In the middle of the meal

10) A side effect *not* associated with Sinemet is:

   a) Dyskinesia

   b) Cramping

   c) Hallucinations

   d) Ringing in the ears

11) Parkinson's disease results from a degeneration of dopamine-producing cells in the part of the brain called:

   a) Cerebellum

   b) Vastus lateralis

   c) Carotid body

   d) Substantia nigra

12) Which of the following is *not* a symptom of Parkinson's disease?

   a) Small handwriting (micrographia)

   b) Soft voice (hypophonia)

   c) Sialorrhea (excessive drooling)

   d) Paralysis

13) Which of the following is *not* a dosage strength of Sinemet?

   a) 10/100

   b) 35/100

   c) 25/100

   d) 25/250

14) When patients are experiencing dyskinesias throughout the day, it probably means:

   a) They don't take enough medicine

   b) They are in need of a medication adjustment

   c) Their diet does not contain enough protein

   d) They are definitely not getting enough exercise

15) Dyskinesias are best described as:
   a) A rhythmic shaking or quivering of a body part appearing exactly as a tremor
   b) An abnormal involuntary movement which may appear as dancing, writhing, or jerking
   c) Very slow movements
   d) All of the above

16) Strategies of coping with Parkinson's disease include all of the following *except:*
   a) Learning more about the condition
   b) Informing family and friends that you have the condition
   c) Attending support group meetings
   d) Masking the condition totally by medicine adjustment and keeping your condition undercover

17) Proper dietary considerations include all of the following *except:*
   a) Avoiding excessive intake of high protein foods
   b) Including high-fiber food choices
   c) Lower-protein foods during the day for maximum medication response
   d) Limiting fluids to only 2 glasses of water per day

18) Constipation can be managed by all of the following *except:*
   a) High-fiber breads and cereals
   b) Exercise and walking
   c) Fresh fruits and vegetables
   d) Vitamins

19) Patients should drink at least:
   a) 1 glass of water per day
   b) 3 glasses of water per day
   c) 6–8 glasses of water per day
   d) 2 glasses of water and 2 glasses of juice per day

20) Which of the following statements about PD is *false*?
   a) There are specific blood tests to diagnose PD
   b) PD symptoms vary and likewise the disease course is somewhat unpredictable
   c) "On" and "off" are terms that describe a person's function at any given moment
   d) Successful management of PD requires a long-term commitment from the patient, family, and health-care team.

AnswerKey: 1)a; 2)a; 3)c; 4)d; 5)d; 6)b; 7)d; 8)c; 9)a; 10)d; 11)d; 12)d; 13)b; 14)b; 15)b; 16)d; 17)d; 18)d; 19)c; 20)a

Chapter Eight

Help for the Caregiver

Until now, the information in this book has been written directly to the patient; the word "you" almost always referred to the person suffering from Parkinson's disease. In many ways, this focus is appropriate, since the goal of therapy for the PD patient is to maintain physical independence for as long as possible. The patient should accept primary responsibility for achieving that goal by learning as much about PD and its treatment as possible.

Nevertheless, there is usually a "power behind the patient," so to speak, someone whose love and support go a long way in making possible a healthy and active life for the patient. In this chapter, "you" refers to the remarkable person known as the caregiver, someone whose own needs and desires often get lost among those of the patient.

You know who you are. Most of you are married to men or women who have been diagnosed with Parkinson's disease. Some of you are daughters or daughters-in-law. Others are sons or close friends. In any case, you're the one who accompanies the patient to the doctor, learns the ins and outs of this complex disease, and helps organize the household to accommodate the patient's needs. You're the one who must watch as the person you love loses some of the physical and emotional verve and vigor he or she once had to a degenerative brain disease.

The role of a caregiver is one to be proud of. There is joy and fulfillment to be found in the help you give to your spouse, parent, or child. But the role is also a taxing one, often filled with stress, frustration, and loneliness. In this chapter, we'll discuss how to balance the needs of the patient with your own. We'll explore some of the practical ways to physically help the patient. Finally, we'll outline the many available options for alternative care: the help of family and friends, adult day care, and, as a last step, entering the patient in a full-time nursing facility.

Who Are the Caregivers?

Although you may feel terribly alone in your situation, you are not the only caregiver in America. You have as fellow travelers the families and friends of the one million Parkinson's disease patients living in the United States today. In addition, millions of women and men of all ages care for others with chronic illnesses with permanent impairment, such as rheumatoid arthritis, heart disease, multiple sclerosis, and stroke.

Most people think that nurses and nursing homes are the primary providers of care for the chronically ill. In reality, however, the vast majority of all long-term care is provided by family members. Of the 4.4 million older Americans who needed long-term care in 1982, for instance, only 1 million lived in institutions. And of those living at home, 85 percent were aided by their families. Who are these stalwart, dedicated people? According to a study conducted by the Wilder Foundation, caregivers have the following characteristics:

- Seventy percent are the primary caregiver.
- One-third are the sole caregiver.
- Seventy-two percent are women.
- Among men, husbands and sons are the most common caregivers.
- Most caregivers are spouses. When a spouse is not available or able, a child, usually a daughter or daughter-in-law, becomes the caregiver.
- Among older caregivers who are spouses, nearly half report that they are concerned about their own health.
- One-third of family caregivers are employed and have employment and parental responsibilities in addition to their caregiving duties.

- Eighty percent of caregivers provide care seven days a week for an average of four hours per day. In instances of severe impairment, including advanced Parkinson's disease, many caregivers provide over 40 hours per week of assistance.

Parkinson's Disease and the Family Dynamic

As you no doubt have already discovered, the diagnosis of a chronic illness—no matter which member it strikes or who becomes the primary caregiver—can throw an entire family for an emotional loop. Adult siblings of the patient come face to face with their own mortality and vulnerability. Adult children are forced to become more independent of, and responsible for, their parents, perhaps

A Special Word About Women Caregivers

Although an equal number of men and women suffer from Parkinson's diseases, over two-thirds of the caregivers are women, including those who care for PD patients. There are many reasons for this discrepancy, including the fact that caregiving has always been a "traditional" women's role. In Parkinson's disease there is the added factor of age: men tend to die at a younger age than women, leaving their spouses alone. The care of a widow with Parkinson's disease is likely to fall to her daughter or daughter-in-law, just as it did in Margaret's case in Chapter Four.

Today's woman, no matter her age, has learned to become a consummate juggler. She is a wife, mother, homemaker, employee, employer, daughter, and, ultimately, primary caregiver. Not only may she care for the chronically ill in her immediate family, but she may feel an obligation (or be pressured) to care for her parents, parents-in-law, and secondary relatives as well. It is not uncommon for a young woman, divorced, working full time, and raising her children alone, to take on the responsibility of caring for her mother or father as well.

If you are a woman—married or single—taking care of someone who is chronically ill, you're likely to be under particular stress, stretching yourself in too many different directions. Read this chapter carefully, and take to heart the suggestions for reducing stress and bolstering your self-esteem.

for the first time. Young children and grandchildren are confused and frightened about what is happening to their loved one. The patient's spouse is forced to reevaluate his or her own life plan in view of the disease and its effects on the family's finances and lifestyle.

It is no wonder, then, that any tension or underlying problems within the family may be exacerbated by a diagnosis of a chronic illness, at least for a time. Although we all want to believe that our families would immediately pull together in a crisis, this isn't always the case.

"I'll never forget my 25-year-old sister's reaction to all of this," recalls Rosemary, the 33-year-old saleswoman diagnosed with PD whom you met in Chapter Four. "Although she seemed supportive, she began making all kinds of demands on my parents, especially my mother. She wanted them to find her a new apartment; she cried about her boyfriend; she borrowed money. Subconsciously, I think she was really trying to take up all my parents' energy so they wouldn't have any for me. And I wasn't much better. My needs and fears were so enormous, I'd end up pushing my mother constantly to do things for me—even things I could do for myself."

This pattern of dysfunctional behavior continued for a number of months, until Rosemary's mother confronted both of her daughters with the situation. "She made us see how hard all of this was on her. We kind of snapped out of it after that. Now we're closer than ever. In fact, my sister is helping me a lot, taking some of the pressure off my mother."

As difficult as sibling and parent-child relationships may become, even more stress is placed on the patient's marriage. If you're the spouse of a Parkinson's disease patient, it's likely that you feel pulled in a hundred different directions. First of all, it's probably up to you to help the rest of your family cope with the effects of the diagnosis. In addition, the patient—your husband or wife—is leaning on you for both emotional and physical support.

Even as you begin to feel more and more like Atlas carrying the weight of the world upon your shoulders, it is your spouse, the patient, who is the object of attention. With the best of intentions, everyone—from doctors and nurses to your family and friends—focuses on the patient's day-to-day physical and emotional health.

When Your Parent or Child Comes to Live with You

Although most caregivers are spouses of PD patients, others of you have a single parent with Parkinson's disease or two parents who are both ill and it has become your responsibility to care for them. Or perhaps it is your adult child who suffers from the disease and counts on you for physical, emotional, and perhaps financial help.

Eventually, the disease may progress to the point where the patient can no longer live on his or her own. You may decide at that point that the patient should move in with you and your family. Needless to say, the family dynamic will undergo considerable emotional change as each member comes to terms with a different household routine and structure. Before you enter into this situation, you and your family should all sit down together and discuss the changes and the new responsibilities that will exist if this occurs.

Among the many practical questions that should be addressed are:

- Will the parent have his or her own room? Who will be responsible for cleaning it and doing the laundry?
- What measures will you take to respect each other's privacy?
- Can the patient stay alone when family members go to work?
- Who will drive the patient to the doctor's office or stay home when needed?
- Who will be responsible for giving medications?
- How will the family handle degenerating health problem such as incontinence or dementia?
- Will extra help be needed at home? If so, who will pay for it? Can the family handle the extra expenses involved?

Again, although your first instinct may be to say, "Things will take care of themselves," it is far better to discuss these issues *before* the patient moves in with you. That way, each member of the family, including the patient, will understand—and have time to accept—what is expected of him or her. This will help to avoid resentment and confusion after the patient has arrived.

Even when major issues have been settled and family roles have been assigned, it is imperative that the lines of communication remain open. Both the patient and other family members must feel able to voice their opinions and emotions freely. It is especially important for the patient to know that he or she can disagree or make reasonable demands without fearing that the family will reject him. Indeed, as difficult as it may be at times, each family member should try to accommodate the changing needs of the patient with love and acceptance. In many ways, the love and acceptance are as important to the patient as medical therapy.

Unfortunately, they forget (and you might, too) that your life has been as disrupted as your spouse's.

Most couples affected by Parkinson's disease are nearing the age of retirement, and no matter which spouse is the patient, both of their lives will change, perhaps dramatically. In a "traditional" relationship, the wife has stayed home while the husband worked. In this case, a wife who has spent most of her adult life raising the children and tending to the household has looked forward to these years as a time to pursue her own interests, lead a more independent life, and perhaps spend time traveling alone with her husband. Now that her husband has been diagnosed with PD, however, it appears that to some degree she'll have to become a caregiver all over again. Depending on the severity of the disease at diagnosis and its subsequent rate of progression, her dreams of increased independence will be limited.

A husband in this age group has probably worked all his life hoping for an exciting retirement. When his wife is diagnosed with a potentially debilitating disease like PD, he may have to care for someone he thought would be a companion on his adventures. Although in most cases the disease will not prevent a patient from traveling, there will be limitations and special considerations. In some ways, this adjustment is more difficult for the husbands of PD patients. Unlike most women, most men have to *learn* to be caregivers, a daunting prospect for many.

Younger marriages, too, are deeply affected by the diagnosis of a chronic illness. Two-income families, in which both spouses need to earn a paycheck in order for the family to be financially solvent, are now the norm in today's society. If one spouse becomes chronically ill and unable to work, how will the family manage financially? If there are children involved and the disease is moderate or advanced, how can the well spouse possibly take care of the kids, tend to the physical needs of the ill spouse, and work at the same time?

None of these questions can be answered the same way for everyone. It is important, however, for you as a caregiver to recognize these stresses and strains before they affect your own emotional and physical health. Keep in mind that, as described in Chapter Six, both the patient and other family members will go through various stages of coping. Although you'll be trying to help them deal with their feelings, you must also allow yourself to experience the same range of emotions.

Do marriages or families crumble over Parkinson's disease? Some do, but usually only the ones that were weak before the diagnosis of PD. The strong ones have a chance to become stronger and closer than ever before. Sustaining good relationships among healthy families is hard enough. When one member becomes chronically ill, even more time and effort must be invested.

If your family is showing signs of dysfunction, it is important for you to find a family therapist or a member of the clergy to help all of you cope in a more healthy way. In addition, try to talk with the spouses and families you meet at support group meetings. They have firsthand knowledge of the struggles you face.

The Patient-Caregiver Partnership

As discussed in Chapter Six, the best doctor-patient relationship is a partnership, one based on mutual respect and equal involvement in the treatment of the disease. So, too, is the most satisfying and successful relationship between patient and caregiver.

Depending on the patient's symptoms, it is likely that you'll become—if you haven't already—part speech therapist, part exercise trainer, part nurse, and part emotional coach. As the disease progresses over the years and the patient's mobility is further restricted, you'll find yourself helping him or her get dressed, use the bathroom, eat, make telephone calls, write letters—in effect, you'll become his or her arms and legs.

To become so intimately involved in another person's most private life is difficult for both you and the patient, even if—or perhaps especially if—the two of you are married. Even with the best of intentions on both of your parts, the relationship can become distorted and dysfunctional.

"I went to a luncheon held by our support group," explains Emily, the 67-year-old wife of a mildly affected PD patient named Joe. "I sat across from a couple, Chris and Agatha. Agatha was severely disabled and Chris was an absolute saint with her. I had seen them at meetings quite frequently and watched how patient and tender he was with her. He helped her in and out of her wheelchair, adjusted her scarf, made sure she sat up straight so she wouldn't drool or look terrible. My husband's symptoms are pretty mild and really didn't need my help most of the time. I wondered if I could ever be as attentive with him when the time came."

Emily's feelings changed at the luncheon, however. "What upset me was the way Chris not only helped her but literally took over for her. He answered for her when someone spoke to her, he ordered lunch for her, and when she wanted to eat potato chips with her sandwich, he told her she couldn't, that they weren't good for her. It was like he was speaking to a child. I vowed then and there never to treat my husband as less than an adult, with his own opinions and rights."

The line between helping and dominating your spouse is a fine one, and you must be vigilant of crossing it. Otherwise, the vicious spiral of dependence described in Chapter Six can result: the more you do for the patient, the less the patient will be able to do for himself or herself. This kind of "learned helplessness" has two unfortunate results. First, the patient's self-esteem will fall in direct proportion to his or her decreasing abilities and sense of self-reliance. Second, eventually your role as caregiver may completely overwhelm you. Performing every act and looking after every detail of the patient's life will leave no time for meeting your own needs and desires.

Under some circumstances, relying on the patient to tell you when your help is needed is sufficient. However, if the patient is feeling overly sorry for himself and depressed, you may end up doing too much for him, risking overdependence. Conversely, if he overestimates his abilities, then you'll do too little for him, risking his safety.

Instead, force yourself to step back and judge the patient's abilities objectively. If you like, ask the doctor or physical therapist about what the patient is able to *safely* do on his or her own. Then, working in partnership with the patient, decide where your help is most beneficial and where it is interfering with the patient's independence. For instance, if your husband's main problem is with his balance and he needs to take your arm during your evening walk, then of course feel free to help him in that way. But if he still has strength in his arms and hands, don't feel that you have to cut his meat or tie his shoes for him.

Perhaps the best thing you can do for your loved one with Parkinson's disease is to encourage independence in all things physical and emotional, even if it at times frightens you. For instance, even if you worry that your husband will be embarrassed about his tremor, encourage him to keep his weekly golf dates. Even if people ask your wife to repeat herself because her voice is so slow, don't speak for her in conversation. Even if your son has fallen down in the past, encourage him to perform his exercises every day (in a safe space and with the aid of a physical therapist, if necessary).

Above all, for both your sakes, try not to let the disease become the total focus of either your relationship or your individual lives. If you're married, for instance, don't neglect your sex life. If you're siblings, enjoy the same activities you did before one of you became ill, even if it means arguing about what movie to see or where to go for dinner. In essence, keep your relationship as equal and natural as possible for as long as possible, even as you face the challenges of the disease together.

How to Lend a Helping Hand

First of all, consider yourself a full-fledged member of the health-care team. Take the time to learn about the disease in general, and then ask the physician to tell you how the disease specifically affects your partner. Depending on your partner's symptoms, you may want to consult other health-care professionals such as physical and speech therapists. It's important for you to feel confident about your skills both in day-to-day activities and in emergency situations.

One way that you can assist in an unobtrusive but supportive way is to exercise *with* the patient every day or every other day. If your partner is in a relatively mild stage of disease, you can do more adventurous things together—bicycle, jog, or cross-country ski. Of course, a good long walk is a less taxing but equally health-ful alternative. Later, when the disease is more immobilizing, help the patient by putting him or her through a full range of motions. Ask a physical therapist to show you how to slowly but firmly stretch and exercise your partner's arms, legs, and torso when he or she no longer feels able to do so.

As the person closest to the patient, it's up to you to keep on the lookout for balance and gait problems. Many patients don't want to admit that they can't live exactly as they once did. As discussed in Chapter Six, this kind of denial is, in many ways, very helpful. It keeps the patient active and optimistic. On the other hand, it can lead to dangerous falls and injuries. If you notice that your partner is no longer able to maneuver as well as before, you may want to consider ordering adaptive aids and/or reorganizing the furniture to accommodate the patient's needs.

If your partner has problems with speech, you'll want to avoid the well-meaning but undermining habit that Emily noticed between Chris and Agatha: answering questions directed at the patient or otherwise communicating *for* the patient. Instead, when you're alone with your partner, work on the speech therapy suggestions described in the A to Z Guide. If low volume is the problem, prompt the patient to speak louder by standing at a distance from him and asking him to "shout" at you. If he slurs his words, remind him to exaggerate their pronunciation. Initiating speech is difficult for many PD patients; if your spouse has this problem, allow him or her ample time to get started without interrupting.

Obviously, there are literally hundreds of ways to help your part-ner cope with the many challenges of Parkinson's disease. If the patient is severely disabled, for instance, you may have to apply the tips and treatments described in the A to Z Guide yourself.

Avoiding Spouse Burnout

The task you have undertaken—that of providing loving and sen-sitive care for someone suffering from Parkinson's disease—is not an easy one. At the same time you are struggling to help your loved one manage with the disease, your financial resources may be dwindling, your "friends" may desert you as the disease takes up more and more of your time, and your own feelings of anger, frustration, and guilt may be getting ready to boil over.

If you're not careful, you'll experience what is known as burn-out, a form of emotional and physical exhaustion associated with a total commitment to and immersion in a job or cause. To avoid burnout, you've simply got to remember to *take care of yourself first*. To help you evaluate how you're handling your role as care-giver, take the time to fill out the accompanying Caregiver Sanity Worksheet.

Accept Your Frustration: Discuss your concerns with the patient, health-care team, and your support group. Keeping your emotions bottled up in order to "spare" the patient may only end up back-firing: you will become more and more stressed, irritable, and unhappy.

Be Assertive: Make sure that your opinions and needs are heard, understood, and respected by your spouse and the rest of the health-care team.

Get Enough Rest: If you're unable to sleep well at night because the patient disturbs you, consider getting separate beds or bed-rooms. Take any opportunity available to grab a nap or relax.

Get Plenty of Exercise: At least three times a week, get 30 minutes or more of vigorous aerobic exercise. (See Chapter Five for more details.)

Learn to Manage Stress: As covered in Chapter Seven, The A to Z Guide to Symptoms and Side Effects, your well-being, physical and emotional, is directly linked to the amount of stress in your life and your ability to deal with it in healthy ways. Deep breathing exercises, meditation, biofeedback, and many other techniques may help you release the tension and stress in your life. Exercise is also a very good stress-reliever.

Caregiver Sanity Worksheet

The most *stressful* thing about caring for someone with Parkinson's disease is _____

_____

The most *irritating* thing about caring for someone with Parkinson's disease is _____

_____

The most *exhausting* thing about caring for someone with Parkinson's disease is _____

_____

The most *rewarding* thing about caring for someone with Parkinson's disease is _____

_____

The most *frightening* thing about caring for someone with Parkinson's disease is _____

_____

Please answer the following questions "yes" or "no"
Do you get 5–6 hours of uninterrupted sleep most
   nights?   _____
Can you arrange to be alone for some portion of every
   day?   _____
Is there someone you could/would call for help at
   2 A.M.?   _____
Is there one friend or family member who could/would
   loan you money if you were in financial trouble?   _____
Is there anyone in your life who fully understands the
   day-to-day trials you experience?   _____
Can you arrange one or two breaks from caregiving at
   least twice a year?   _____
Two steps I will take in the next month to simplify my life:

_____

_____

Eat Well: Proper nutrition is as important to your health as it is to the patient's. If the patient is on a special diet, you may have to cook separate meals for yourself.

Accept the Support of Your Support Group: Nothing can match the healing power of empathy and compassion, two qualities found in abundance at your local APDA support group. (See Appendix I for more details.)

Be Selfish with Your Free Time—what little there may be of it! At least once a week, treat yourself to a special lunch out, a softball game with your friends, a manicure, a movie. Make sure you maintain your own interests or develop new ones that have nothing whatsoever to do with your spouse or with Parkinson's disease. You may even want to take on a part-time job or volunteer activity.

Most important of all, *recognize when you've done all you can.* Deciding to seek additional help (as discussed below) can be difficult. Consider talking with a social worker or a family therapist to help clarify your needs and make appropriate choices.

Finding Respite Care

At some point, you're going to need more sustained and regular help to care for your partner—and that time should be *before* you become physically ill or emotionally overwrought. As soon as you notice that you no longer have any time for yourself or are feeling constantly exhausted, take some of the burden off your shoulders. There are a number of options available to you. Take advantage of one or more of the following:

Family and Friends: If you have told them often that you can handle everything, many people may now take you at your word: No longer does your daughter offer to take her father away for the weekend to give you time alone. Neither does your neighbor suggest that she do your grocery shopping when she does her own, thereby giving you time to take a nap.

Nevertheless, chances are that they would still be happy to help you out—if you'd only ask. As difficult as it may be for you, pick up the phone and call, keeping in mind that your health and the patient's are in jeopardy if you don't.

Home Care: If transportation is a problem or if the patient is severely disabled, you can hire health-care professionals—physical therapists and nurses, among others—to come to your home on an hourly, daily, or weekly basis. This allows the patient to get the needed care as well as giving you a little time on your own. Depending on your insurance and/or government assistance, some or all of this home care may be covered. Contact your local Council for the Aging or Parkinson's disease support group or Information and Referral Center for more information (see Appendix I).

Adult Day Care: For an afternoon every week or for eight hours every day, you can take your partner to a center where he or she can find companionship, necessary health and personal care, exercise, and more—all at a reasonable price. Sound too good to be true? According to recent statistics, there are more than 1,000 adult day-care centers throughout the United States. Adult day-care centers may be sponsored by a PD support group, a hospital, church, senior center, or other local agency.

Adult day-care centers offer many services, including medical help, assistance with self-care procedures, and physical therapy. The patient also has a chance to meet people suffering from the same or a similar condition, often gaining emotional support and a renewed sense of optimism and purpose.

An adult day-care center also can serve as a bridge between living alone or within a family setting and placement in a long-term, nursing-care facility. Many adult day-care centers are affiliated with or even housed in a nursing home.

Long-Term Residential Care: At some point, you may no longer be able to care for the PD patient. Perhaps your husband's or wife's condition has become so severe that constant medical care is required. Or perhaps your own health is impaired and you can no longer perform the daily care routines for the PD patient.

One option is to place the PD patient in a long-term care facility, commonly known as a nursing home. About 6 percent of the over-65 population and 21 percent of the over-85 population live in such facilities. For many people, the single most difficult decision they ever make is to place a parent or a spouse into a nursing home. The decision almost always feels wrong. Nevertheless, although you and your family may be frightened by the thought of sending the patient away, a nursing home—staffed by caring, qualified people with expertise in coping with the needs of advanced PD patients—will provide your loved one with a safe and reliable residence.

Basically, there are three different kinds of long-term care facilities: *medically necessary care*, which in many ways approximates hospital care; *skilled nursing facilities*, which offer 24-hour nursing care and other health services for the convalescent and/or chronically ill; and *intermediate care facilities*, which offer nursing care as needed, health services, and personal assistance in daily living. Some nursing homes are affiliated with retirement communities, allowing a patient to live independently in a separate apartment for as long as possible, then transferring to the nursing home itself. (The cost of these services, and how to pay for them, is covered in more depth in Chapter Nine.)

Within these general categories, there are many different types of nursing homes. Choosing one that best suits your loved one will require some legwork on your part. It is never too early to start researching your options; some of the best nursing homes have extensive waiting lists. The factors to consider when evaluating a facility are:

- *Location.* No decision about location should be made until all members of the family have been consulted. Which relatives will be visiting most often? Is it accessible by public transportation? How close are other medical facilities?
- *Level of care provided.* Ask the patient's physician to evaluate the patient's level of disability to see where he or she fits into the nursing home categories mentioned earlier.
- *Quality of care.* The best way to find a good nursing home is to check with your local Council on Aging, your state department of elderly affairs, or your local Parkinson's disease support group.

- *Costs.* Find out what the costs are and the prices of extras such as laundry, doctors' visits, and medications. Make sure that the facility is Medicaid-certified. Keep in mind that the nursing home wants to be sure that you have private funds available to pay for the cost of care for a number of months, up to nine months in some cases. Therefore, you almost never get an answer to your question about bed availability until the nursing home gets an answer about who will pay. (See Chapter Nine for more details.)

Once you've placed your partner in the facility, it's up to you and other family members to make sure that he or she is receiving appropriate care. If you are concerned about any facet of care, talk to a nurse, nursing director, administrator, the doctor, social worker, or physical or occupational therapist. If you're frustrated in your effort to talk with the staff or are frustrated in getting the care you want for the patient, call your local or state long-term care ombudsman.

Planning Ahead

"Ten years ago, when my husband was diagnosed with PD, everyone—including the doctors—told us to take things one day at a time," recalls Marianne. "We did just that and are we sorry for it now. We coped day to day just fine, but we never made any long-range financial plans. Now that my husband has lost his job, we've got to scramble to find out about insurance and disability. His condition seems to be getting worse and worse, and I'm having to imagine what will happen when I can't take care of him anymore. I just don't know what we'll do."

Marianne and her husband aren't alone. Because PD often progresses quite slowly, planning for a future in which the patient is severely disabled is an unpleasant, and therefore often postponed, task. However, it's never too early to think about setting up a financial plan. In the next chapter, you'll learn about your options for insurance and other forms of financial aid, as well as tips on protecting your assets and life savings.

Chapter Nine

Planning Your Financial Future*

At the turn of the century, the average life expectancy in the United States was 47 years. As we reach the twenty-first century, life expectancy has increased to 75 years and people commonly live much longer. The fastest-growing segment of our society is the population over 65. That's perhaps why we are seeing more cases of Parkinson's disease now than when James Parkinson first defined the syndrome.

The longer we live, the more susceptible we become to illnesses that may incapacitate rather than kill us. Although some people in their 20s, 30s, and 40s suffer with Parkinson's disease, most patients with PD as well as with other debilitating illnesses such as stroke and heart disease are in their 60s and 70s.

No matter what your age, however, once you are struck with a chronic illness, your financial stability is in jeopardy. The United States is the only industrialized country without a national health insurance program. Millions of people—even some who are employed—have no health insurance to begin with; others with chronic illness may lose their health insurance when they are no longer able to work. There are very few safety nets for those of us who become chronically ill. As a society and as individuals we are facing some fundamental questions in our struggle to care for the increasing numbers of Americans who cannot afford the spiraling costs for medical care.

* Adapted with permission from *How to Protect Your Life Savings from Catastrophic Illness and Nursing Homes: A Handbook for Financial Survival* (Boston: Financial Planning Center, 1991), by Harley Gordon.

To keep your head above water financially after a diagnosis of PD, you must plan carefully, even though the financial aspects of long-term disability are often the last thing you and your family want to talk about. Upon diagnosis, you and your spouse may suffer, at least temporarily, from shock and denial. Even those family members with a little emotional distance may think it distasteful, insensitive, or even crass to talk about money when someone has just been diagnosed as having a long-term, potentially debilitating disease like Parkinson's.

Spouses are emotionally devastated by the thought that their life partner may one day be incapacitated. If the patient is a primary wage earner, even the short-term financial questions are difficult to ponder. How long will my husband/wife be able to keep working? What about medical insurance? Will he or she be eligible for a pension? Can we expect disability payments from the employer? The long-term questions are even more painful. What will happen if the family can no longer care for the patient? How can we afford to pay for nursing home care? Will we lose our life savings to this illness?

No matter how hard it is to think about these issues, there is no question that an honest discussion is in order, since the longer you wait to make decisions, the more likely it is that you'll run into serious financial difficulties. In order to receive Social Security benefits, for instance, you must apply in advance and often must wait a number of months before your benefits arrive. If nursing home care is required and you haven't protected your assets, a lifetime of work and savings can be wiped out within a matter of months.

Financial planning, with all of its intricacies, is far beyond the scope of this book. This chapter will serve only as a kind of mini-primer in organizing your financial future. First, you'll learn about the need for advance directives: wills, living wills, and powers of attorney. The various types of federal and local financial and health insurance available to you are also discussed. Then, in the second part of the chapter, you'll find out how to protect your family's assets from being attached by Medicaid to pay for your care in a nursing home, should that become necessary.

To start, you should conduct a thorough examination of your financial health. The essential part of that analysis is your personal "net worth." To calculate your net worth, estimate the following:

1. Your yearly net income, whether from employment, Social Security, or both
2. Your house equity (its present estimated market value minus any outstanding loans you have on it)
3. Values of any stocks and bonds
4. Savings accounts and savings bonds, certificates of deposit, IRAs, and other bank accounts
5. Additional real estate holdings, minus any outstanding loans
6. Any other major assets
7. Then calculate your outstanding loans and other forms of indebtedness

With this information, you can begin to prepare your financial plan. It is highly advisable that you seek the aid of a lawyer or financial planner, preferably one who specializes in the financial needs of the chronically ill. Some suggestions for finding a lawyer are listed at the end of this chapter.

Filing Advance Directives

As unpleasant as the thought may be, we will all die one day. Before we die, many of us will also become incapacitated and unable to make our own financial or medical decisions. Preparing for those eventualities is essential, for both your family's financial future and your own peace of mind.

The basic documents you need to prepare your estate are

1. Living will
2. Durable power of attorney for both health care and finances
3. Last will and testament

A *living will* is a directive to your physicians to avoid the use of life-support equipment or other extraordinary measures to sustain your life. Because medical science has made it possible for humans to be kept alive by technology for an indefinite amount of time, many people are now choosing the right to die rather than be sustained in this manner. The result is the living will, now recognized as a legal document in all states.

However, it should be noted that the use of living wills is not widespread. It is estimated that only about 15 percent of Americans across the country have signed living wills or chosen a health-care proxy. Many doctors are not yet comfortable discussing what they view as a disturbing subject, and therefore they do not suggest or encourage their patients to set up such a directive. In addition, because the legality of living wills is still being challenged, decisions are made—by the family or the doctor—that countermand the patient's wishes in about 25 percent of all cases.

For these reasons, many people are appointing a health-care proxy (a person who is legally designated to make decisions about treatment and medical care should you become impaired) or signing a durable power of attorney, a person whom the patient trusts to uphold his or her wishes.

Power of Attorney

A power of attorney is a legal instrument that gives to another or others the right to handle your financial affairs. Typically, a person will create a power of attorney to give another the right to have access to a bank account or to sell stock on his behalf. The person given this responsibility does not have to be an attorney.

A *regular* power of attorney usually gives specific and limited powers like the ones mentioned above. It usually does not have an expiration date but ceases the minute you become incapacitated. The moment the agreement is signed, you lose control of your assets to your power of attorney.

A *durable* power of attorney is exactly the same as a regular power of attorney, except that it remains valid even if you become incapacitated. A durable power of attorney allows someone to take care of such financial chores as paying your bills, buying and selling your securities, cashing your checks, selling your house, opening or closing bank and brokerage accounts, and collecting money due you. It can also be very effective in planning to protect assets that otherwise would have to be spent on a nursing home. If you become ill and are unable to handle your assets, the person or persons to whom you assign the power of attorney will be able to transfer your assets into their own names, making them inaccessible to Medicaid.

In some states, a durable power of attorney for asset management and a durable power of attorney for health care can be prepared as one document. In other states, two separate documents must be prepared. Some people prefer having two different people accept these very different responsibilities; that is a personal matter between you and your family.

Warning: Giving a power of attorney is giving away control. It is not advisable to do this unless absolutely necessary. Instead, draw up the document and give it to someone who is trustworthy to hold until it is needed. Instructions should be given about how and when it will be used.

If your state allows it, consider putting two people on the power of attorney so that there are checks and balances—two people will have to agree on how to manage your affairs. In addition, consider a *springing* durable power of attorney. This instrument is valid only when you become incapacitated—a judgment made by your family, doctor, and attorney—unlike a regular or durable power of attorney which becomes effective the moment you sign.

Last Will and Testament

Everybody needs a will, no matter what his age, value of assets, or state of health. A will is simply a legal document stating your wishes for the settlement of your estate (everything you own) after your death. A will is the best way to (1) determine the distribution of your personal belongings and assets; (2) provide for family needs, including naming a guardian for minor children; (3) plan wisely for taxes, helping your heirs minimize estate and income tax on what they inherit; and (4) make charitable contributions. *Only by having a will can you be sure that your wishes will be carried out after you die.*

To be sure that your will is valid and that your estate is financially protected, you need the help of a lawyer and, depending on the value of your estate, a financial adviser such as an accountant or bank trust officer.

Make sure you update all of your legal documents on a regular basis. The biggest mistake lawyers and financial advisers make is to forget to inform their clients that most financial institutions will not accept certain documents after a period of time. There is no set policy on when the instrument becomes "stale." A power of attorney or a living will is only as good as a person's or institution's willingness to accept it. Update by rewriting it (if only by changing the effective date) at least every two years.

Now that you've made a financial analysis of your assets and have considered advance directives such as wills and powers of attorney, you should begin to think about your more immediate future.

Are You Still Working?

If you have PD but are under 65 years of age and are still working, you have a number of pressing financial issues to consider. As discussed in the Employment section of the A to Z Guide, it is illegal for an employer to fire a person because of an illness or disability—as long as you're able to do your work. If your employer is concerned about your abilities, offer to let him or her speak to your physician if further clarification is necessary.

At the same time, or perhaps even before meeting with your employer, take stock of your company's policies regarding disability and pensions. In addition, reevaluate its health insurance plans in consideration of your illness. Ask your personnel department to discuss these matters with you, but until you receive legal and financial advice from a qualified attorney, do not sign any agreements concerning your termination, pension, or disability.

If you're enrolled through your company in a group health insurance program such as Blue Cross/Blue Shield or a Health Maintenance Organization (HMO), stay covered for as long as possible. Most company health plans allow you to maintain the policy for 18 months after leaving your job—no matter why you leave—allowing you time to arrange for health insurance on your own.

Are You Unable to Work?

If you're unemployed, without medical insurance, and you have Parkinson's disease, it may be difficult to find a private, affordable insurance company to cover you, especially since you'll want a major medical policy that will cover most of the significant medical expenses that you have now and may have in the future. If you have trouble finding coverage, ask someone in your PD support group or an APDA Information and Referral Center for recommendations.

If you are retired, cannot afford private insurance, and/or need further assistance in meeting your expenses, there are government-sponsored options available to you, namely Social Security, Medicare, and Medicaid.

If you are over the age of 62, you are eligible to collect *Social Security retirement benefits*, a government insurance program that you paid for during your working life through deductions made from your paycheck. Your benefits are calculated through a complex formula based on your total earnings over your working lifetime. (To check your Social Security status, request form SSA-7004 from the Consumer Information Center, Dept. 55, Pueblo, CO 81009, fill it out, then send it to your local Social Security office. It will tell you how much money you've earned in your life, and how much in Social Security benefits you are eligible for.)

In addition to retirement benefits, the Social Security Administration (SSA) offers *Medicare*, a hospital and voluntary medical insurance program available to all people over the age of 65, who are receiving Social Security retirement benefits. Medicare provides basic protection against the costs of both hospital insurance (including inpatient hospital care and home health care) and medical insurance (including physician's services, medical services and supplies, home health care, and outpatient hospital services). Those over 65 who are not eligible for Social Security may still purchase Medicare coverage. Check with your local SSA office.

Be aware, however, that Medicare *does not* pay all of the above costs: it will pay only for the first 60 days of hospital costs (minus a deductible); after 60 days, you will pay a certain amount ($89 a day in the state of California, for instance) and Medicare will pay the rest. As for medical expenses, Medicare pays 80 percent of approved medical charges (with a $75 deductible paid by you).

For those under the age of 65 who are disabled, Social Security offers another form of Medicare called Social Security Disability Insurance. There is no financial means test for eligibility; you can be wealthy or poor to receive SSDI. After receiving SSDI support for two years, the disabled person becomes eligible to receive regular Medicare benefits whether he or she has reached the age of 65 or not.

Supplemental Security Income and Medicaid

Someone of any age who does not qualify for Social Security or whose total available income from all sources (including Social Security retirement benefits and/or SSDI) does not meet a certain level (which varies from state to state) may apply for assistance from another agency called Supplemental Security Income. SSI is a basic cash benefit program for the aged and disabled whose income falls below a certain level. In Massachusetts, that level was $536 per month for a single disabled person in 1991.

If you are eligible for SSI, you automatically qualify for *Medicaid*. Medicaid is a medical assistance program to help certain needy and low-income people of any age. Medicaid pays for a variety of medical needs, including inpatient and outpatient hospital services, physicians' services, some home health-care services, and long-term care in a nursing home. Your total income and assets must fall below a certain level for you to be eligible for Medicaid. Under certain circumstances, someone over the age of 65 can be eligible for *both* Medicare and Medicaid.

Negotiating your way through the maze of federal, state, and private assistance programs is no easy task. Depending on your particular needs and disabilities, you may benefit from a state-funded program more than a federally funded one. It is best to get help from a professional with experience in these matters, either an attorney or a social worker. Your local support group or American Parkinson's Disease Association Information and Referral Center will be able to recommend someone in your area.

Protecting Your Assets in the Event of Long-Term Care

Although only 15 percent of the chronically ill enter a long-term facility, that number ends up being 1 million people every year, many thousands of whom are advanced Parkinson's disease patients. While it may be a difficult step to take, you and your family should contemplate the possibility of your entering a chronic care facility sometime in the future. As you'll see, waiting too long could mean losing your hard-earned life savings.

As described in Chapter Eight, nursing homes provide three basic types of care:

- Medically necessary care (which in many ways approximates hospital care), for which Medicare will pay.
- Skilled nursing care, which provides patients with continuous care and assistance by nurses and other professionals.
- Intermediate care for those who need help with everyday routine daily activities.

Medicare or other types of medical insurance plans will not pay for skilled nursing care or intermediate care, since they are considered custodial (not medically necessary) care. The yearly cost for this kind of care can run as high as $65,000 in the Northeast and on the West Coast to $25,000 in the South, Southwest, and Midwest.

Many people mistakenly think that there is some insurance or other system that will pay these bills. In fact, however, there are only three sources to pay for long-term nursing home care:

- *Cash.* At a national average cost of $35,000 a year for nursing home care, a recent American Association of Retired Persons (AARP) poll found that an average family's life savings would be wiped out within nine months.
- *Medicaid.* No one likes to apply for public assistance. It is one of the great ironies that the very system that older Americans have struggled for years to avoid is for many the only means to pay for nursing home care. That holds equally true, of course, for younger persons.
- *Nursing home insurance.* Insurance companies are beginning to offer plans that will pay certain amounts toward daily custodial care for a period of years. These policies may be the right answer for those who fear the financial consequences of nursing home confinement but who want to maintain control of their assets for as long as possible.

Unfortunately, most of the nursing home policies currently available aren't worth the paper they're written on. They are often filled with so many restrictions, exceptions, and limitations that one recent survey conducted by Congress found that less than a third of policies ever pay a dime!

But that doesn't mean that nursing home insurance is a bad idea. In fact, in certain cases, it may make some sense. Unfortunately, buying nursing home insurance is as confusing and perilous as buying a used car. Since a good policy for a person in reasonably good health, at age 65, averages between $1,200 and $2,000 a year, do not enter into a contract without first consulting an attorney or financial adviser well versed in the ins and outs of this type of insurance.

The Basics: Understanding Medicaid

Under the current system, there are two factors that determine eligibility for public assistance: assets and income. We'll discuss assets first.

Assets

The definition of assets is: *everything you own that has value*. That definition seems simple enough. Medicaid, however, divides assets into three categories: countable assets, noncountable assets, and inaccessible assets. Don't try to make sense out of why a particular asset falls into one category and not another. No one ever said that the Medicaid program was rational. In fact, it sometimes seems that Medicaid is as confused as we are in trying to figure out what they will force us to spend before Medicaid benefits will begin and what they will let us keep.

Countable Assets. These are the things that Medicaid requires you to deplete in their entirety before financial assistance is available. They include

- Cash over $2,000 (in most states)
- Stocks
- Bonds

- IRAs
- Keoghs
- Certificates of deposit
- Single-premium deferred annuities
- Treasury notes and treasury bills
- Savings bonds
- Investment property
- Whole life insurance above a certain amount (depending on what state you live in)
- Vacation homes
- Second vehicles
- Every other asset that is not specifically listed as non-countable is included in this list

The things listed above are in jeopardy when catastrophic illness strikes. In order to qualify for Medicaid, the applicant must in effect be BANKRUPT.

Noncountable Assets. Believe it or not, these items can be worth hundreds of thousands of dollars, but Medicaid so far has chosen not to count them in determining eligibility. They include

- A house used as a primary residence (in most states this includes two- and three-family homes)
- An amount of cash (usually $2,000, depending on your state)
- A car
- Personal jewelry
- Household effects
- A prepaid funeral
- A burial account (not to exceed $1,500 in most states)
- Term life insurance policies (as opposed to whole life) which have no cash surrender value. Life insurance is generally divided into two groups: whole life and term. Whole life has a cash value which increases the longer you hold the policy. Although the insurance lapses when you stop paying, you receive cash value back. This is called the policy's surrender value. Term insurance, on the other hand, never builds up a cash value, but is worth only the face amount on the policy and then only when you die. Coverage stops when you stop pay-

ing. Most states allow you to keep unlimited term insurance when applying for Medicaid, but only a limited amount of whole life insurance.

Inaccessible Assets. These are countable assets which have been made unavailable to Medicaid. To put it bluntly, if you can't get them, they can't get them. Assets are made inaccessible by

1. Giving them away
2. Holding them in Medicaid trusts (see below)
3. An involuntary situation in which the person who owns the assets is too incapacitated to gain access to them

Medicaid Trusts

In order to protect the assets that Medicaid is able to attach, you may want to hold them in what is called a Medicaid trust. There are two kinds of trusts: revocable and irrevocable. The difference between the two is that the first can be changed after it is set up, the second can't.

A *revocable trust* is a legal instrument that you set up to hold assets. There must be at least one trustee and one or more beneficiaries. A trustee is simply the person who makes the decisions for the trust. The beneficiary is the person who gets the benefit of the assets in the trust. Since you make the trust, you make the rules that the trustee must follow. If you don't like the trust, you can change it or do away with it. That's why it is called revocable. A revocable trust also acts as a will. The rules you make can include who gets your money and under what conditions after you die. While you are alive you receive the benefits. This kind of trust is useful in protecting your house, but it will *not* protect countable assets.

An *irrevocable trust*, like a revocable trust, is a legal instrument that you set up to hold assets. Like a revocable trust, there must be one or more trustees and one or more beneficiaries. The definitions of a trustee and beneficiary are the same as above. You can make the same rules. The difference is that once you've made the rules, you can't change them. By making it irrevocable, you give up the power to modify or do away with the trust. Simply put, you lose control.

The only trust that will protect countable assets is an irrevocable trust but *only* one that limits the amount of discretion of the trustee(s). This is the trust that qualifies as a Medicaid trust.

Congress passed a law that took effect in 1986 restricting the use of an irrevocable trust. The law states that if you set up an irrevocable trust, name yourself as a beneficiary and give the power to your trustee to give you all, some, or none of the income and assets, Medicaid will assume that your trustee will make all the income and principal available to you and thus the nursing home. It doesn't matter that your trustee can say, "I have the power to refuse to give the nursing home any money." Medicaid won't accept that explanation and will force you to spend those assets before covering your expenses.

The trust has to be set up in such a way as to limit the power of the trustee. If the trustee has no power to give you the assets, but only to hold them, Medicaid can't get them—they will not have to be spent before Medicaid will cover your nursing home or other medical expenses.

For example, here's an irrevocable trust that *doesn't* protect assets: A husband and wife set up The ABC Family Trust. They name their son as the trustee and themselves as beneficiaries. They give the trustee the power to give them all, some, or none of the principal and income. The day that a parent/beneficiary goes into the nursing home is the day a thorough appraisal is taken of the couple's assets. Since they gave discretion over the assets and income to the trustee, Medicaid assumes that the trustee will use his full discretion and make the assets and income available to the parent. In other words, the assets are considered countable, available, and therefore subject to division just as if they weren't in trust. Until they are spent, Medicaid will not cover your expenses.

An example of an irrevocable trust that *does* protect assets: A husband and wife set up The ABC Family Trust with the same trustee and beneficiaries. This time they don't give any power to the trustee to give them assets, only the power to hold them in trust while they generate income. The day that a parent goes into the nursing home is the day that an assessment is made of their assets. (This assessment is known as a "snapshot.") However, this time the assets in the trust are not in the snapshot because the trustee cannot make them available to the parent. Therefore, the assets do not have to be spent before Medicaid coverage begins.

WARNING: There are thousands of Medicaid qualifying trusts that were set up prior to 1986 which were made invalid by the law Congress passed that year. Today, none of these trusts will protect assets even though they were legal and effective when set up. If your trust was established before 1986, be sure to contact your attorney to make the appropriate changes.

Remember, in defining noncountable assets, specifics vary from state to state. Be sure to check with your state Medicaid office to see how assets are classified in your locale. Also, regulations may change through legislation, so be sure to check with your local welfare agency when planning or filling out an application for Medicaid.

The Spousal Impoverishment Act

The Spousal Impoverishment Act (SIA) supposedly protects a stay-at-home spouse (the person not going into a nursing home) by allowing him or her to keep certain amounts of assets and income.

As of October 1, 1989, Medicaid treats marital assets this way:

Step 1—Medicaid determines the day when a spouse goes into a nursing home or medical institution.

Step 2—Medicaid requires that the couple list all their countable assets regardless of whose name they are in, who earned them, or how long they've been in either's name.

Step 3—Medicaid takes a snapshot, a picture of the combined assets on the day the spouse goes into the nursing home or medical institution.

Step 4—The stay-at-home spouse is then allowed to keep one-half of the total amount of the assets in the snapshot, but not less than $13,296 or more than $66,480 annually. (These numbers go up every year.)

For example, Curtis, who has had PD for 15 years, is going into a nursing home on June 1. He and his wife, Helen, have total assets of $20,000, $15,000 of which is in his IRA. Medicaid will take a snapshot of the couple's combined assets on June 1. Helen will be allowed to keep one-half of $20,000. Since half of $20,000 is $10,000, she will be allowed to keep $13,296, the *minimum* the state allows her to keep. If Curtis and Helen had $150,000, Helen would not be allowed to keep half ($75,000) but only $66,480, the *maximum*.

To make matters a little more confusing, although the general principles here are consistent across the board, the dollar amounts may vary from state to state. The law allows each state to set the amount that the stay-at-home spouse may keep between a minimum of $13,296 and a maximum of $66,480. Here's how that works:

Your state may decide to raise the floor on the amount that a stay-at-home spouse may keep of their joint assets. Rather than a floor of $13,296, your state may allow $40,000. What happens in our example when the floor is raised to $40,000? Helen would be allowed to keep the entire $20,000, and Medicaid pays for Curtis's care in toto.

An application for Medicaid is usually not made on the day that the spouse goes into the nursing home. Whether the spouse will be able to qualify is determined by using the four-step method described above.

If assets have to be spent by the institutionalized spouse in order to qualify, the application for Medicaid may not take place for months. Regardless of what the total assets are on the day he applies, the stay-at-home spouse's share will always be determined on the day of the snapshot—the day the patient enters the nursing home.

For example, Joel and Esther have combined countable assets of $100,000 at the time Esther goes into a nursing home on January 1. The snapshot is taken on January 1. Joel's spousal share (the amount he is allowed to keep) is $50,000. Unless Esther buys noncountable assets or otherwise protects her money, she will have to spend $48,000 on her care ($50,000 minus $2,000, the maximum assets she can keep).

But let's say that Joel applies for Medicaid for his wife when there is $70,000 left of countable assets. All Esther would have to spend is $18,000 before she is eligible for Medicaid. Why? Because Medicaid goes back to the financial snapshot taken on January 1, the day Esther went into the nursing home. Joel's share at that time was $50,000. This amount deducted from $70,000 leaves $20,000 that Esther will have to spend. She is allowed to keep $2,000 of that amount. It is important, then, to protect as many of your assets as possible before applying for Medicaid.

Income

Income is all the money you receive from any source. Like countable assets, it is in jeopardy should you need to apply for Medicaid when you or a loved one enters a nursing home. The money may come from one or a combination of the following:

- Social Security
- Interest and investments
- Trusts
- Rental units
- Help from family members
- Pensions
- Annuities

Income eligibility is quite simple. In most states, if the person who is going into the nursing home has monthly income that exceeds the nursing home bill, he pays the nursing home directly. If that person's monthly income is less than the nursing home bill, Medicaid has him give it to the home and Medicaid makes up the difference. Most, if not all, of your income, regardless of where it comes from, for whatever reason you get it, will have to go to the nursing home.

Most states allow single people to hold back:

- a personal needs allowance (anywhere from $30 to $70 per month, depending on the state)
- a home maintenance allowance (if the patient is planning to go back home to live)
- a monthly premium to pay for medical insurance

Income rules do not apply to the stay-at-home spouse. He or she is free to continue working and keeping the salary and other monthly income (like Social Security). In addition, the state usually allows the spouse to keep her half of the assets that generate income, such as dividends, rent, etc.

The law requires states to set a specified amount that the stay-at-home spouse may keep from total joint income. As of October 1, 1989, the minimum was $815 per month, the maximum was $1,500. The states have discretion in setting the amount within those limits. The well spouse has the opportunity to increase the state-set amount if she can show that her housing expenses are unusually high.

For example: Dennis and Eleanor's only income is $1,200 a month in Social Security. Of that, $1,000 is the husband's, $200 is his wife's. If Dennis goes into a nursing home, he will be allowed to make the following deductions from his $1,000:

- a personal needs account
- the premium for his insurance policy that pays the deductibles on his Medicare policy
- $615 monthly to supplement is wife's $200 a month, since the minimum she is provided from the spousal income is $815.

Remember, Eleanor's own personal income is unaffected. If she is working, all her salary remains hers. She does not have to make a contribution to Dennis's nursing home expense. Please note, however, that 20 states now impose a limit, or cap, on how much income a nursing home patient can earn each month and still be covered by Medicaid—*no matter how much the nursing home care costs.* In 18 states, that limit is $1,221. Therefore, if Dennis earned $1,222 a month, he would be ineligible for Medicaid coverage even if his nursing home bill was $2,500 a month. In that case, it would be up to Eleanor to make up the difference. Please check with your local Medicaid office to see if your state has instituted income capping.

How to Protect Assets When There's Time to Plan

One of the good things about Parkinson's disease is that, although it is a degenerative disease, it is slowly degenerative. Most patients lead healthy and active lives for some years after diagnosis before they are incapacitated. Nevertheless, it is important for financial planning to take place as soon as possible, especially if you are elderly when you receive your diagnosis. In this section, you will find out how to protect your assets when you have time to plan. Please note, however, that there *are* things you can do to protect your finances in an emergency. (For more information, see *How to Protect Your Life Savings*, by Harley Gordon.

The key to protecting your assets is knowing what assets and income are in jeopardy and what the critical deadlines are for transferring them. In the preceding section, we identified which assets and income are in jeopardy.

Our goal is to take countable assets (those that have to be spent to zero) and make them either noncountable (and therefore protected) or inaccessible, which means that Medicaid can't force you to deplete them before covering the costs of your care. Now we will look at the options available to people in different situations.

Remember: The key to protecting assets when you have time to plan is understanding the rules about disqualification. When a transfer of a countable assets is made to the inaccessible category, the person making the transfer is disqualified for a period of months. Read and memorize the following rule: *If you transfer countable assets for less than fair market value within 30 months before applying for Medicaid or going into a nursing home or a medical institution, it is presumed that you did it to have Medicaid pay the expense of institutional care.* Therefore, Medicaid will not cover the costs of nursing home care until those assets are depleted or until 30 months have passed since the transfer of assets took place.

For example, Sam is a widower PD patient whose balance problems have steadily worsened. He now feels that full-time residential care will become necessary within a year. On January 1, 1990, he transfers all his savings ($50,000) to his son. He enters the nursing home a year later, on January 1, 1991. Since he gave his money away within 30 months of being institutionalized, he will not qualify for Medicaid until either 18 months has passed (30 months minus the 12 months that passed between the date of transfer and his entry into the home) or he has spent all the transferred money on paying his nursing home bills.

If assets are to be protected, it is imperative that a transfer be made at least 30 months before the day the applicant goes into the nursing home or applies for Medicaid.

This is especially important if the nursing home resident went in before October 1989 (when the disqualification period was increased to 30 months for all states). Since he would be subject to his state's old law, there may be severe penalties for applying for Medicaid within the old disqualification time. Never apply for Medicaid benefits until after the entire disqualification period (old and new) has passed.

At this point, we have covered the general principles involved in protecting assets. Now let's get down to specifics. There is no single course of action that best suits every situation. There are different ways to protect your assets depending on whether you want your spouse, offspring or parents, siblings, nieces and nephews, aunts and uncles, to be the beneficiaries.

For our purposes, we'll concentrate on what happens in the case of a married couple, one of whom has Parkinson's disease and is considering entering a nursing home. Again, this example certainly won't apply to everyone reading this book, but it should give you an idea of the general principles involved.

John and Suzanne Andrews—our couple—have just found out that John has Parkinson's disease. Below is a quick financial sketch of the Andrews family:

Name:	John and Suzanne Andrews
Age:	both 65
Assets:	house $150,000 (jointly held, no mortgage)
	savings (joint) $50,000 (includes wife's inheritance of $10,000)
Insurance:	husband has two insurance policies, a whole life policy with a face value of $10,000 and a cash surrender value of $2,000 and a term policy worth $25,000
Income:	joint, from savings $4,000/year
	Social Security: husband $650/month
	wife $300/month
Health:	husband, early Parkinson's disease
	wife, good
Family:	two adult children, Bill (with whom they don't get along) and Susan (with whom they are close)

The goal is to take countable assets and move them to the noncountable or inaccessible column (see *The Basics: Understanding Medicaid*, above, for definitions). Here is how the assets would be categorized at the time of the Parkinson's disease diagnosis before steps are taken to protect them:

Noncountable	*Countable*	*Inaccessible*
house	savings $50,000	none presently
term policy	whole life policy	

Now, what happens when John and Suzanne *don't* plan. If assets remain in the countable column, they will have to be spent on nursing home care, subject to the Spousal Impoverishment Act, before John qualifies for financial assistance. If these assets are transferred to the inaccessible column within 30 months of going into a nursing home, Medicaid presumes he is trying to hide these assets. He will have to either spend these assets or wait until 30 months have passed after the transfer of assets before he can be covered by Medicaid.

Please note: In reviewing how the Andrewses' assets are divided, you will notice that his term life insurance policy is noncountable and therefore can be kept. Not so with his whole life policy, since the face value, not the cash surrender value, exceeds a certain amount. It is suggested that Mr. Andrews transfer ownership of the policy to one of the children in order to make it inaccessible.

Here's what will happen if the assets remain exactly as they appear above: On the day John enters the nursing home, Medicaid will take a snapshot of the couple's assets regardless of whose name they are in. Since the countable assets were not shifted to other categories, Suzanne will be allowed to keep only a specified amount. That figure is arrived at by applying the somewhat confusing formula mentioned earlier: Suzanne may keep no less than $13,296 or one-half of their combined total assets up to a limit of $66,480, whichever is greater.

Looking at the Andrewses' chart, we see that their joint funds are $50,000. Half of that is $25,000. Since $25,000 is greater than $13,296 and less than $66,480 she is allowed to keep $25,000.

Here's what happens if their savings account is $15,000 instead of $50,000. One-half of $15,000 is $7,500. Because $7,500 is less than $13,296, she gets to keep the greater amount ($13,296), since that is the *minimum* the law allows.

What would have happened if their savings account had been $200,000? One-half of that amount is $100,000. Because $100,000 is greater than $66,480, she gets to keep only $66,480 since that is the *maximum* the law allows.

If you are feeling confused, you're not alone. These rules seem arbitrary even to professional financial planners. To add another layer of accounting, individual states are allowed by law to raise the amount that the stay-at-home spouse may keep.

Let's say, for example, that the Andrewses live in a state where the minimum amount Suzanne can keep is $40,000. Our chart shows total countable assets of $50,000. One-half of $50,000 is $25,000. Because the floor is now $40,000, however, Suzanne gets to keep not one-half (or $25,000) but $40,000 of their $50,000 in joint assets.

Now, let's say that the couple had $150,000 in joint assets. One-half is $75,000. Because $75,000 is more than the ceiling of $66,480, she would keep only $66,480. In this case, the floor ($40,000) is not used.

Now let's see what happens when John and Suzanne *do plan*. Because John received his diagnosis when he was at a fairly early stage of Parkinson's disease, he and his wife have more than the required 30 months in which to protect their assets before they need to apply for Medicaid. Assets may be protected (made inaccessible) by:

1. Giving them away to the spouse
2. Giving them away to offspring
3. Holding them in trust
4. An involuntary situation where the applicant is too sick to gain access (not applicable in the Andrewses' situation)

After examining each option, we will see which is best suited to this specific situation.

Option 1: Giving Away Assets—One Spouse to the Other

A good example of how fast Medicaid law is changing is the

November 1989 revision of the regulation covering spousal transfer of assets. Prior to that time, the only spouse who was prohibited from transferring assets was the one being institutionalized. As long as the stay-at-home spouse had countable assets in her name for at least 30 months, she was free to transfer them without penalty even if the transfer occurred the day before the snapshot (the assessment made by Medicaid the day the spouse enters the nursing home).

John, for instance, could have taken his name and Social Security number off all the countable assets. The account would then be in the name of his wife only, or if she wished, she could add a son or daughter as a coholder.

Let's say 30 months have passed from the day of the transfer. Under the old law, if Mr. Andrews were institutionalized, his wife would have been free to transfer the assets to the children so long as this was done before the day of the snapshot. Since Suzanne was not being institutionalized, her assets (those in her name for at least 30 months) could be transferred without penalty.

However, the option of giving all the countable assets to the healthy spouse for the purpose of protecting them from Medicaid is no longer viable. The law *after November 1989* puts the Andrewses in a new position. Suzanne has had all the countable assets in her name for at least 30 months. Her husband is going into a nursing home tomorrow. Under the new law, if she tries to transfer the assets to her children, Medicaid will consider the transfer as if her husband had made it: He will be disqualified for 30 months or until the countable assets are spent. Therefore, the option of giving all the countable assets to the healthy spouse for the purpose of protecting them from Medicaid is no longer viable.

Option 2: Giving Away Assets—To the Offspring

Here's a little wisdom to ponder: Never give your assets to your children unless you are absolutely, positively willing to stake your life on the belief that they will give them back or make them available to you when you ask.

Here's what you want to avoid:

The children spending them because they "thought they were a gift"

Your son's or daughter's spouse (whom you never liked in the first place) getting your assets in a divorce

Your son or daughter losing the money in a bad business deal

A rule of thumb in determining whether your offspring should be chosen to hold and protect your assets: If you have to think more than one-half of one second before you answer "yes," forget the whole idea. On the other hand, if you do have a close and trusting relationship with your offspring, you can enlist their help in protecting your assets.

Option 3: Holding Assets in Trusts

As you learned in the section entitled "Medicaid Trusts," above, there are different kinds of trusts to consider. Here are two examples using the Andrews family:

An irrevocable trust that *doesn't* protect assets:

The Andrewses set up the Andrews Family Trust, naming their children as trustees and themselves as beneficiaries. They give the trustees the power to give them all or some or none of the principal and income. The day that John goes into the nursing home is the day that a snapshot is taken of their assets. Since they gave discretion over the assets and income to the trustees, Medicaid assumes that the trustees will use their power and make the assets and income available to the parents. In other words, the assets are considered countable and therefore available, subject to the Spousal Impoverishment Act.

An irrevocable trust that *does* protect assets:

The Andrews set up the Andrews Family Trust with their children as trustees and themselves as beneficiaries. This time, however, they don't give any power to the trustees to distribute the assets, only the power to hold the assets in trust while they generate assets and income for them. The day John goes into the nursing home is the day the snapshot is taken of their assets. However, this time the assets in the trust are not in the snapshot because the trustees cannot make them available to their parents. Therefore, Medicaid will cover the costs of the nursing home costs. However, Medicaid may force John and Suzanne to spend their joint income to pay nursing home bills.

If the Andrewses decide to use a trust, here are their options:

- Plan A: They can establish an irrevocable trust like the second example above.
- Plan B: They can establish an irrevocable trust like the second example above but naming a third person as a beneficiary and giving the trustee power to distribute funds to that third person. For instance, they establish the Andrews Family Trust, making it irrevocable. They name themselves as beneficiaries along with a third person, such as their daughter, Susan. They name a fourth party as trustee and give him control over the assets. The trust allows the trustee to give only Susan the principal at any time, never John and Suzanne. The Andrewses can get money only through Susan, the third beneficiary. If either John or Suzanne goes into a nursing home, the principal will be protected, since the trustee never had discretion to give principal to either of them.
- Plan C: The Andrewses can establish a revocable trust naming John and Suzanne as beneficiaries but specifying that the trust becomes irrevocable if either one of them goes into a nursing home or has a long-term illness.

Which plan is best?

Plan A means that the Andrewses give up full control of the assets well before John goes into the home. This is the same as giving them away. Also, with this type of trust, they can't get their principal.

Plan B still means that the Andrewses give up full control of their assets. However, the trustee can give the assets to a third person, who in turn could make them available to the Andrewses. Of course, during the time that John is not in the nursing home, the

Andrewses will have to get their assets through that third party-(daughter Susan in their case, but it could be a close friend or other relative). If John does go into a home, the trustee can still get money to Suzanne by using the above method.

However you slice it, this trust takes control away from the Andrewses. If the Andrewses do not feel comfortable with giving this power to a relative or close friend, this option doesn't work for them.

Plan C means that the Andrewses' assets are countable and available to Medicaid for 30 months. Why? Because revocable trusts don't protect countable assets. The trust in Plan C becomes irrevocable only when there's a long-term illness or nursing home confinement. At that point, 30 months must expire before assets are protected. This plan is useful only for people with a great deal of money who can easily afford to pay privately for 30 months. The Andrewses can't.

Which plan, then, is best for this couple? If a trust is to be used, Plan B is best because it protects the assets while still making them available through a third person. The key is that the third person *must* be trustworthy.

So, then, which option is the best one for the Andrewses? Option 2, Plan B: Holding money with a third person as beneficiary is the best alternative other than giving the money outright to the children.

Under such a plan, here is how the transferred assets line up:

Noncountable	*Countable*	*Inaccessible*
house	0	whole life insurance policy now owned by Susan
term policy		assets in trust

The Andrewses represent just one of the many possible relationships and financial situations. Your own situation may be quite similar. Just as likely, however, you fit into a far less "traditional" living situation: You're a widow with children, an independently wealthy single man, a young woman with no assets but a good job, or a healthy adult child with not one, but two, chronically ill parents.

Finding the Right Financial Attorney

As you can see just from this short analysis of one couple's financial situation, planning for your own financial future may be a complicated affair. Indeed, even if you have few assets or are still working full time, there are a number of questions that may be best answered by an attorney well versed in the needs of the chronically ill.

The practice of Medicaid law, for instance, is a very specialized field. Few lawyers can speak its language fluently.

Here are some suggestions for finding an attorney with expertise in this field.

- Contact the National Academy of Elder Law Attorneys at 655 N. Alvernon Way, Suite 108, Tucson, Arizona 85711. This organization is made up of lawyers who specialize in problems of the elderly.
- Call your local Council on the Aging or its equivalent for referrals.
- Speak to the social worker at your area hospital. Many have dealt with nursing home placement and are familiar with attorneys who work in the field.
- Speak to your doctor. If he treats many Parkinson's disease patients, he is likely to be able to refer you to someone with experience in financial planning for the chronically ill.
- Perhaps the best place of all to find a lawyer or accountant to help you through the maze is your local Parkinson's disease support group or Information and Referral Center (see Appendix I).

Here are some suggestions on how *not* to find an attorney:

- Don't choose an attorney from an advertisement. Anyone can call himself an expert.
- Don't rely on the local bar association referral service. Few if any have a category that deals with this subject. If they deal with it at all, they lump it together with estate planning. Estate planners do not necessarily understand all the contingencies of a chronic illness, especially Medicaid law.

Parkinson's Disease and Your Future

If you work to maintain careful financial plans, scrupulous medical care, and an optimistic spirit, there is every reason to believe that you and your family will successfully cope with the challenges of Parkinson's disease. Nevertheless, you no doubt hope that a cure or a treatment to stop the progression of your disease will be found before too long.

In the next chapter, you'll learn about current research being conducted by scientists throughout the country seeking to solve the mystery of Parkinson's disease.

Chapter Ten

Parkinson's Disease and the Future

THE BRAIN, still known as medicine's "last frontier," is today the focus of some of the most exciting new research in this altogether remarkable age of science and medicine. We have learned more about the way the brain functions and misfunctions during the past thirty years than in the centuries of research that preceded them. Luckily for those of you reading this book, Parkinson's disease, perhaps more than any other single brain disorder, has benefitted most from this focus.

When James Parkinson first defined the disease that now bears his name in 1817, patients had little hope. Their brains, drained of dopamine, would no longer create the synapses required for proper human movement and posture. They were doomed to lives of immobility and deformity. Even thirty-five years ago, little could be done to keep a Parkinson's disease patient active and healthy. Today, effective drug therapy has dramatically changed the outlook for PD patients. With care and diligence, most parkinsonians can continue to work and play for many years.

Nevertheless, if you have been diagnosed with PD or love someone who has the disease, these extraordinary advances in understanding the syndrome and in treating it are not enough. You, like the one million other American PD patients and their families, want more. You want a way to stop your brain cells from dying. You do not want to have to take effective—but toxic—drugs several times a day, every day, for the rest of your life. You want a cure.

Hundreds of scientists in labs across the country are diligently working to help you. Funded by pharmaceutical companies, government grants, and with the aid of the four national Parkinson's disease organizations, these scientists, separately and in concert, are looking at several different avenues of therapy and remedy.

Drug Research

By far, the most promising and exciting new drug treatment is selegiline or deprenyl, marketed under the name Eldepryl. As you may remember from Chapter Four, selegiline is an MAO B inhibitor: it blocks the action of the enzymes responsible for breaking down excess chemical transmitters. There is also some reason to believe that this drug retards the progression of the disease itself, acting in some way as a neuroprotector, shielding brain cells from premature degeneration. If indeed this is so, an eventual cure for Parkinson's disease may lie in finding ways to increase the efficacy of selegiline or similar drugs so that a complete halt to the degeneration of brain cells occurs.

A second avenue of drug research is focused on the dopamine agonists, the drugs that work to directly stimulate the nerve cells in the striatum without the need for the neurotransmitter dopamine. If the synapses that create proper movement can occur without dopamine, it means that the patient with PD does not need to take as much levodopa. A new agonist called cabergoline, currently under investigation, may be given on a once a day basis and may provide more long-acting relief of symptoms.

Why does it take so long for a drug to become available for use? In the United States, the route from chemistry lab to the pharmacy is a long and complicated one. The Food and Drug Administration strictly controls which products can be sold, demanding extensive scientific data on two important issues: proof that the drug indeed helps patients with a given disorder and proof that it is not dangerous. For anti-Parkinson drugs, the process may be particularly slow, since serious side effects of the drugs may not present themselves for several months or even years.

Surgical Treatment

The most controversial treatments for Parkinson's disease involve brain surgery to repair or replace the brain cells lost to the disease process. Surgery for the treatment of Parkinson's disease was first performed in the 1930s. Various operations were carried out in which some region of the cerebral cortex was removed or fibers deep in the brain were cut. The idea was to damage the motor pathways just enough to diminish tremor or rigidity without causing other impairment. The results, as you might imagine, were unpredictable and often negative.

As medical science advanced, surgical techniques improved. One of the most important new procedures, first developed in the late 1940s, is called stereotactic surgery. This technique involves the use of a long needle which is lowered into the brain through a tiny hole made in the patient's skull, thus alleviating the need for opening the skull and exposing the fragile brain to the outside environment. The direction and depth of the needle are calculated by computer with incredible precision.

At first, surgeons concentrated on a small bundle of tissue located deep in the cerebral hemisphere in the forebrain known as the thalamus. The thalamus is believed to be a relay station for all the sensory messages that enter the brain. Using electrical currents or other information, surgeons stereotactically operated on the thalamus, a procedure known as a thalamotomy. Some patients benefitted dramatically from this surgery; others did not. Moreover, many patients found that the symptoms returned after many months or years, often in a different part of the body than the original symptoms. In addition, although the mortality for this procedure was relatively low, there were risks involved—namely, the danger of a stroke if the needle injured a blood vessel.

Once the efficacy of levodopa therapy was established, most surgical procedures were discontinued. However, in some selected patients with severe tremor, a thalamotomy performed by an experienced surgeon is a good option. Recently, scientists are focusing on the surgical *implantation* of cells in the brain. These cells come either from the patient's own adrenal gland or from brain tissue derived from fetuses. Highly controversial and with as yet unknown long-term effects, tissue implantation remains at the forefront of current PD research.

• *Adrenal transplantation* involves taking cells from the adrenal glands (located on the top of each kidney) and implanting them in the brain, usually in the caudate nucleus or the putamen, both parts of the basal ganglia that receive messages from the substantia nigra. Adrenal tissue is chosen because it is can produce dopamine outside the brain.

In the United States, about 250 adrenal tissue transplants have been completed since 1987, with only a few appearing to have had lasting clinical benefit to the patients. The consensus among many scientists is that while the adrenal surgery helps some patients, even dramatically, the results are inconsistent and unpredictable. In addition, the complication rate is relatively high, especially in debilitated patients with advanced disease, who are more likely to submit to the surgery. Until the factors, considered below, which govern tissue survival are better understood, many scientists are against continuing with adrenal surgery. Recently, however, the combination of adrenal surgery with the infusion of trophic (growth) factors that promote cell survival have been successfully performed in animals.

• *Fetal tissue transplantation* involves taking cells from the brain of a fetus and implanting them in the brain of a Parkinson's disease patient. Once there, some scientists believe that these cells would enhance and possibly restore dopamine production by leading to the actual growth of new dopamine cells.

Success with fetal work in humans was reported in number of countries, including Sweden, Great Britain, the United States, China, Cuba, and Mexico. Because the tissue is derived from fetuses that have been aborted, however, fetal research is controversial. The use of aborted fetuses to treat any disease, including PD, has been limited because the U.S. government has banned all funding related to fetal research, and most medical and research facilities depend on federal grants. Today, only two centers, Yale University School of Medicine and the University of Colorado, currently use fetal tissue, relying entirely on private funds to pay for the research.

Apart from the political controversy, there are a number of medical issues surrounding both adrenal and fetal implantation. Most scientists believe that the variability in outcomes—with a few patients improving dramatically while others don't—results from the fact that scientists are unable at this point to properly identify those cells that will have the best effect in the brain. In other words, from exactly what part of the fetal brain do we take the cells or from what part of the adrenal gland? And how do we best prepare the cells for transplantation?

Second, scientists are uncertain as to the optimal location within the brain for implantation of these cells. The caudate nucleus? The putamen? Unfortunately, a trial-and-error approach is inappropriate: There are considerable disadvantages to implanting tissue into more than one site—namely, the increased risk of complications such as strokes and hemorrhage.

Finally, of most interest, is the evidence that certain substances, known as trophic or growth factors, may help nerve cells or parts of nerve cells to grow. Trophic factors are responsible for actually stimulating growth in damaged nerve cells and for promoting nerve cells to connect with each other. Release of trophic factors may be stimulated through a variety of means, including transplanting (into the brain) tissue known to have trophic factors. The trophic factors may permit the transplanted tissue to survive in the brain or may change the transplanted tissue in such a way that it more nearly resembles nerve cells. Alternatively, the trophic factors may cause the surviving but damaged nerve cells in the PD patient to sprout and take over the function of the dead nerve cells.

One way to answer some of these questions is through the growing science of genetic engineering. As incredible as it may seem, research may make it possible—sometime in the future—for healthy, thriving human brain cells to be created in a laboratory setting and implanted in the brain to replace those lost in Parkinson's disease.

With this technique, a line of the patient's own cells (usually a type of cell called fibroblasts), which are found in the brain's connective tissue or glial cells, would be taken and modified so as to function as nerve cells. After the nerve cells are created, it is hoped, they can be transplanted into the brain to function either as substantia nigra cells releasing dopamine or in other as yet unknown ways to create the synapses needed for proper human movement.

Recently, fibroblasts grown from the skin of a parkinsonian rat were separated from the other lines of rat cells by the technique of tissue culture. While the fibroblasts were growing in tissue culture, the genetic material for making the enzyme tyrosine hydroxylase was inserted into the fibroblasts. As you may remember from Chapter Two, the enzyme tyrosine hydroxylase is involved in the chemical process that changes dopa into dopamine. Fibroblasts ordinarily do not produce tyrosine hydroxylase. After the genetic material for making this enzyme was inserted into the them, however, the fibroblasts were programmed to make the enzyme and could change dopa into dopamine, thereby substituting for the missing nerve cells in the parkinsonian brain.

Such remarkable techniques mean that cells could be taken from a readily accessible source, such as the skin, sparing the patient a major operation (such as that required when removing adrenal gland tissue, for instance). The cells could be grown in tissue culture so that an amount sufficient to reverse the patient's symptoms is obtained and, if necessary, the procedure could be repeated. Since the patient's own cells are being used, there would be no problems with the patient's immune system (the body's major defense against foreign tissue) destroying the implanted cells. The technique of genetic engineering is in its infancy. To date, only fibroblasts from rats have been genetically engineered to produce tyrosine hydroxylase. Much will have to be done before genetically engineered fibroblasts can be taken from the skin of humans with PD and implanted into their brains.

In the meantime, however, other research, also involving brain surgery, continues on new methods of delivering dopamine into the brain (other than by administering a drug by mouth or injection). One of these methods involves a surgical procedure to implant encapsulated cells that secrete dopamine. Because the cells are encapsulated, they are protected from the natural body defenses (the immune system) that otherwise would destroy them. The capsules, however, have small pores that permit the dopamine to be delivered into the brain. The encapsulation of cells that produce specific chemical substances and the introduction of such cells into the brain may mean that these techniques can also be applied to other neurological disorders where specific substances have to be delivered.

Staying Ahead

With a little luck and a lot of diligence, one of these futuristic procedures may end up proving to be a cure for Parkinson's disease, perhaps even within your lifetime. Your partnership with your doctor requires both of you to stay as informed as possible about medical breakthroughs such as those mentioned above. In addition, information about how to better cope with the challenges of day-to-day living with Parkinson's disease is offered by doctors and patients in a number of publications and forums, particularly through the national PD associations located in the United States.

In Appendix I, these resources and many others are listed for your information. Take advantage of them and exercise your considerable power to make your life full, active, and rewarding.

Appendix I

Resources for Patients and Caregivers

If you or someone you love has been diagnosed with Parkinson's disease, you may well feel overwhelmed by the many demands of chronic illness. Where should you turn for financial help? Medical advice? Support for your caregiver? Some days it must seem that yours is the only family suffering with the often exhausting demands of chronic illness.

I hope that after reading this book, however, you've learned that thousands of other families join you in your struggle to lead a happy, healthy life. A large community of professionals and peers exists in every part of the country. In every state and in most large cities, organizations and companies exist that can make your life as a Parkinson's disease patient or caregiver easier and more fulfilling. Some of them deal specifically with Parkinson's disease, others with a whole range of related subjects including insurance and legal matters, benefits for retired people, and support for caregivers. Many of them offer material and advice to you at no cost, while others specialize in selling home health-care products and services designed for the disabled. Take advantage of these marvelous resources—they will indeed help you and your family live life to the fullest.

Parkinson's Disease Organizations

Four organizations in the United States and one in Canada offer patients and caregivers information and support and also sponsor scientific research grants, publications programs, medical symposiums, and support groups.

The National Parkinson Foundation. Known primarily for its diagnosis, treatment, and research center in Miami, Florida, this organization was founded in 1957 by the late S. Jay Levey and continues to be supported by Bob Hope, its honorary chairman. Affiliated with the University of Miami School of Medicine, the foundation offers an outpatient treatment facility that attracts patients from all over the country to visit resident neurologists and participate in physical, speech, and occupational therapy. Informational booklets and a quarterly newsletter are available upon request. The foundation has established research centers at Yale University, New Haven, Connecticut; The Graduate Hospital in Philadelphia, Pennsylvania; Vanderbilt University in Nashville, Tennessee; Baylor Medical School in Houston, Texas; University of Southern California and Loma Linda University in Los Angeles, California.

National Parkinson Foundation, Inc.
1501 N.W. Ninth Avenue
Miami, FL 33136
(305) 547-6666

The United Parkinson Foundation. Founded in Chicago in 1963 to keep patients educated about the latest developments in Parkinson's disease research, the UPF sends regular newsletters and other literature, usually free of charge upon request, to interested patients and caregivers. About half of its funds, raised through public donations, are spent on research grants. The UPF also sponsors regional seminars featuring internationally known neurologists and other experts on Parkinson's disease.

United Parkinson Foundation
220 South State Street
Chicago, IL 60604
(312) 922-9734

The Parkinson's Disease Foundation. Affliated with Columbia University, the PDF places primary emphasis on research to find the cause and cure for Parkinson's disease.

Parkinson's Disease Foundation
William Black Medical Research Building
640 West 168th St.
New York, NY 10032
(212) 923-4700

The American Parkinson's Disease Association
60 Bay Street, Suite 401
Staten Island, NY 10301
(718) 981-8001
(800) 223-2732

The APDA has 47 Information and Referral Centers, 80 chapters, and more than 350 support groups located throughout the United States. They can help you find the right neurologist, provide you with booklets and pamphlets that will help you better understand Parkinson's disease, and set you up with the best speech and physical therapists available locally. Many centers offer lectures and/or clinics on a regular basis as well. In addition, these centers can refer you to social workers or lawyers that can help you plan financially.

Perhaps most important of all, each APDA Information and Referral Center will help you connect with a support group in your area. Nothing compares with meeting someone who is going through the same things you are.

Please address all inquiries to the
"APDA Information and Referral Center"
at the following locations:

ALABAMA

BIRMINGHAM

University of Alabama at Birmingham
Department of Neurology
1218 C Jefferson Tower
University Station
Birmingham, AL 35294
(205) 934-9100
FAX: (205) 934-0928

ARIZONA

PHOENIX

Barrow Neurological Institute
350 West Thomas Road
Phoenix, AZ 85013
(602) 285-6652
FAX: (602) 650-7161

TUCSON

1650 East Fort Lowell, Suite 302
Tuscon, AZ 85719
(602) 326-5400
FAX: (602) 694-2727

CALIFORNIA

IRVINE

University of Irvine
Department of Neurology
107 Irvine Hall
Irvine, CA 92717
(714) 725-3500

LOS ANGELES

The Neurosciences Institute
The Hospital of the Good Samaritan
637 South Lucas, Suite 501
Los Angeles, CA 90017-2395
(800) 841-8765

SAN DIEGO

4010 Morena Boulevard, Suite 224
San Diego, CA 92117
(619) 273-6763
FAX: (619) 273-6145

RANCHO MIRAGE

Eisenhower Memorial Hospital
42201 Beacon Hill
Palm Desert, CA 92260
(619) 773-1480
FAX: (619) 773-3105

SAN FRANCISCO

Seton Medical Center
1900 Sullivan Avenue
Daly City, CA 94015
(415) 991-6687
FAX: (415) 991-6024

SANTA MARIA

APDA Young Parkinson's Information & Referral Center
1041 Foxenwood Drive
Santa Maria, CA 93455
(805) 934-2216
(800) 223-9776
FAX: (805) 934-4950

COLORADO

DENVER

Colorado Neurological Institute
300 East Hampton Avenue, Suite 205
Englewood, CO 80110
(303) 781-5788
FAX: (303) 777-4245

CONNECTICUT

NEW HAVEN

Hospital of Saint Raphael
Senior Services
175 Sherman Avenue
New Haven, CT 06511
(203) 789-3936
FAX: (203) 789-4289

DISTRICT OF COLUMBIA

Georgetown University School of Medicine
Department of Neurology
3800 Reservoir Road, N.W.
Washington, DC 20007
(202) 687-5468
FAX: (202) 784-2261

FLORIDA

MIAMI BEACH

Neuromedical Research Foundation, Inc.
1135 Kane Concourse
Bay Harbor, FL 33154
(305) 865-3082
(800) 825-2732
FAX: (305) 866-1844

ST. PETERSBURG

St. Petersburg Sun Coast Chapter
5970 80th Street North, #101
St. Petersburg, FL 33709
(813) 544-2732

TAMPA

Parkinson's Research Corporation
1207 Parilla
Tampa, FL 33613
(813) 968-9557

GEORGIA

ATLANTA

Emory University School of Medicine
1365 Clifton Road, N.E.
Room 5102
Atlanta, GA 30322
(404) 248-5120
FAX: (404) 248-3767

IDAHO

BOISE

St. Alphonsus Medical Center
1055 North Curtis Road
Boise, ID 83706
(208) 378-2369
FAX: (208) 378-2277

ILLINOIS

CHICAGO

Center for Health Aging
St. Joseph Hospital & Health Care Center
2900 North Lakeshore Drive, Room 716
Chicago, IL 60657
(312) 975-3325
FAX: (312) 975-3056

KANSAS

KANSAS CITY

Kansas University Medical Center
Neurology Department, Room 1025 "C"
3901 Rainbow Boulevard
Kansas City, KS 66160-7134
(913) 588-6992
FAX: (913) 588-6965

LOUISIANA

NEW ORLEANS

Hotel Dieu Hospital
2021 Perdio Street, 8th Fl.
New Orleans, LA 70112
(504) 588-3365
FAX: (504) 588-3699

MARYLAND

BALTIMORE

Johns Hopkins Outpatient Center
Department of Neurology
601 North Caroline Street, Room 5065
Baltimore, MD 21287
(410) 955-8795
FAX: (410) 955-6402

MASSACHUSETTS

BOSTON

Boston University School of Medicine
Department of Neurology
720 Harrison Avenue, Suite 707
Boston, MA 02118
(617) 638-8466
FAX: (617) 859-8441

MINNESOTA

MINNEAPOLIS

Methodist Hospital
P.O. Box 650
Minneapolis, MN 55440
(612) 932-5607
FAX: (612) 932-5987

MISSOURI

ST. LOUIS

Washington University Medical Center
School of Medicine
Box 8111, 660 Euclid Avenue
St. Louis, MO 63110
(314) 362-3299
FAX: (314) 362-2826

MONTANA

GREAT FALLS

Montana Deaconess Medical Center
1101 26th Street South
Great Falls, MT 59405
(406) 455-5464
FAX: (406) 455-4969

NEBRASKA

OMAHA

6910 Pacific Street, Suite 104
Omaha, NE 68106-1044
(402) 551-9311

NEVADA

RENO

V.A. Hospital
1000 Locust Street
Reno, NV 89520
(702) 328-1715
FAX: (702) 328-1464

NEW JERSEY

NEW BRUNSWICK

Robert Wood Johnson University Hospital
1 Robert Wood Johnson Place
New Brunswick, NJ 08901
(908) 745-7520
FAX: (908) 753-8856

NEW YORK

FAR ROCKAWAY

Peninsula Hospital
51-15 Beach Channel Drive
Far Rockaway, NY 11691
(718) 945-7079
FAX: (718) 945-6828

MANHATTAN

Hospital of Joint Diseases
Orthopedic Institute, Department of Nursing
301 East 17th Street, Room 1111
New York, NY 10003
(212) 598-6300

OLD WESTBURY

N.Y. College of Osteopathic Medicine
New York Institute of Technology
Old Westbury, NY 11568
(516) 626-6114
FAX: (516) 626-9290

ROCHESTER

The University of Rochester
School of Medicine and Dentistry
Department of Neurology, Room 5-5206
601 Elmwood Avenue
Rochester, NY 14642
(716) 275-3679
FAX: (716) 473-4678

SMITHTOWN

St. John's Episcopal Hospital
Route 25A
Smithtown, NY 11787
(516) 862-3560
FAX: (516) 862-3105

STATEN ISLAND

Staten Island University Hospital
Ambulatory Pavilion, 2nd Fl.
475 Seaview Avenue
Staten Island, NY 10305
(718) 226-6129
FAX: (718) 226-6167

NORTH CAROLINA

DURHAM

Duke South Medical Center
MPDC—Box 3809
Durham, NC 27710
(919) 681-2033
FAX: (919) 660-3853

OHIO

CINCINNATI

University of Cincinnati Medical Center
Charles D. Aring Center
234 Goodman Street
Cincinnati, OH 45267-0520
(513) 558-6770
FAX: (513) 558-5403

OKLAHOMA

TULSA

Hillcrest Medical Center System
3220 South Peoria
Tulsa, OK 74105
(918) 747-3747
FAX: (918) 749-2449

OREGON

PORTLAND

The Oregon Health Sciences University
  Department of Neurology
3181 S.W. Sam Jackson Park Road
Portland, OR 97201
(503) 494-5285
FAX: (503) 494-7228

PENNSYLVANIA

PHILADELPHIA

Clinical Neurophysiology Laboratory, Room 1
Crozer-Chester Medical Center
1 Medical Center Boulevard
Uplands, PA 19013
(215) 447-2911
FAX: (215) 447-6278

PITTSBURGH

University of Pittsburgh
School of Medicine, Department of Neurology
322 Scaife Hall
Pittsburgh, PA 15261
(412) 648-2024
FAX: (412) 648-1239

RHODE ISLAND

PROVIDENCE

Roger Williams Medical Center
Ambulatory Pavilion
50 Maude Street
Providence, RI 02908
(401) 456-2456
FAX: (401) 456-2272

TENNESSEE

MEMPHIS

Methodist Hospital
One Crews
1265 Union Avenue
Memphis, TN 38104
(901) 726-8141

TEXAS

DALLAS

Presbyterian Hospital of Dallas
8200 Walnut Hill Lane, Suite 237
Dallas, TX 75231

(214) 891-4224
(800) 725-2732
FAX: (214) 345-2571

LUBBOCK

St. Mary of the Plains Hospital
4014 22nd Place, Suite 2
Lubbock, TX 79410
(806) 796-2647
FAX: (806) 796-0689

SAN ANTONIO

The University of Texas H.S.C. at San Antonio
Division of Neurology
7703 Floyd Curl Drive
San Antonio, TX 78284-7883
(512) 567-6688
FAX: (512) 567-4659

WASHINGTON

SEATTLE

University of Washington
Division of Neurology, RG27
Seattle, WA 98195
(206) 543-5369
FAX: (206) 685-8100

WISCONSIN

MILWAUKEE

St. Mary's Hospital
2320 North Lake Drive
Milwaukee, WI 53201-0503
(414) 225-8031
(800) 433-4508 (out of state)
(800) 522-0802 (in state)
FAX: (414) 291-1048

General Health Issues

Unfortunately, having Parkinson's disease does not make you immune to
other health problems, such as diabetes, heart attacks, vision problems,

and other diseases. And with or without Parkinson's disease, staying fit and healthy should remain a top priority for each and every one us. Following is a list of national organizations that can provide you with information on wide-ranging health issues.

National Health Information Center
P.O. Box 1133
Washington, DC 20013-1133
(800) 336-4796

This federal agency maintains an up-to-date list of health-related organizations across the country as well as a library of books and pamphlets available to the public for a small fee. It also can provide referrals related to health issues to both professionals and consumers.

Keeping your heart and circulatory system healthy is as important with Parkinson's disease as it is without. The American Heart Association, with branches in every major city across the country, is a font of information about all aspects of cardiovascular health. In addition, the American Medical Association and the National Easter Seal Society also have pamphlets, booklets, and audiovisual material relating to diet and exercise, stopping smoking, and other general health information.

The American Heart Association
7320 Greenville Avenue
Dallas, TX 75231
(214) 373-6300

The National Easter Seal Society
70 East Lake
Chicago, IL 60612
(312) 726-6200

American Medical Association
535 North Dearborn Street
Chicago, IL 60610
(312) 464-5000

General information on prevention and treatment of disease is available from the following organizations; should you want to learn more about CPR and other emergency care procedures, the Red Cross offers classes in many communities. Please note that there are branches of the Red Cross in major cities across the country.

Canadian Council on Social Concern Self-Help Unit
P.O. Box 3505
55 Parkdale Avenue
Ottawa, On K14 461 Canada
(613) 728-1865

Over 200 organizations throughout Canada participate in this self-help clearinghouse, including Parkinson's disease associations.

National Health Information Center
Office of Disease Prevention and Health Promotion
P.O. Box 1133
Washington, DC 20013-11332
(202) 619-0257

American Red Cross
17th and D Streets, N.W.
Washington, DC 20006
(202) 737-6300

Physical fitness is important for everyone, especially those with Parkinson's disease. In almost every town in the country, health clubs and spas, not to mention the good old reliable YMCA, can provide you with a safe environment in which to exercise. Work with your physical therapist and your physician to develop a safe exercise plan for you, and contact the following two organizations if you'd like more ideas on different types of exercise programs:

President's Council on Physical Fitness and Sports
400 Sixth Street, N.W.
Washington, DC 20201

American Alliance for Health, Physical Education and Recreation
1201 16th Street
Washington, DC 20036

The following videotape contains exercises for people with Parkinson's disease and is to be used in conjunction with prescribed medical treatment. Review this program in its entirety with your physician and medical advisers before attempting the exercises.

Health Tapes Inc.
P.O. Box 47190
Oak Park, MI 48237
(800) 521-0334

Personal and Home Health-Care Aids and Products

If you need help in performing day-to-day activities, there are adaptive aids available to make tasks, from getting dressed in the morning to speaking on the telephone to cooking dinner at night, a little easier. Ask for catalogues from the companies below:

Abledata
Adaptive Equipment Center
Newington Children's Hospital
181 East Cedar Street
Newington, CT 06111
(203) 667-5200

Accent on Living
P.O. Box 700
Bloomington, IL 61702
(309) 378-2961

Radio Shack/Tandy Corporation
500 One Tandy Center
Fort Worth, TX 76102
(817) 390-3700

Sears Home Health-Care Catalog
Sears Tower
Chicago, IL 60607
(800) 366-3000

AT&T Special Needs Center
2001 Route 46, Suite 310
Parsippany, NJ 07054-9990
(800) 233-1222

The Recording and Research Center
1245 Champa
Denver, CO 80204
(303) 893-4000 ext. 282

Lifeline Systems, Inc.
One Arsenal Marketplace
Watertown, MA 02172
(617) 923-4141

Lifeline is a personal response system which links you to 24-hour assistance at the push of a button. A small, portable help button is worn on a neckchain or wrist strap or clipped to clothing. If you need help, simply push the button. A Lifeline communication is connected to your telephone line. It sends an automatic call for help when you push your button. For more information, call for their brochure.

Concerns of the Elderly

The financial, legal, and emotional issues that confront the aging—whether healthy or ill—are often quite daunting. A number of organizations have been set up to help you find your way through this confusing maze. One of the best is your state office on aging or elder affairs, which you can find in your local yellow or white pages. Local offices of the United Way can also offer advice and resources to you, free of charge. Other associations specializing in elder affairs include:

American Association of Retired Persons
1909 K Street, N.W.
Washington, DC 20049
(202) 872-4700

The AARP is a membership organization that offers insurance and investment programs, travel information and discounts, and other programs for elders. The AARP also produces a number of publications and audiovisual programs, available to its members.

Commission on Legal Problems and the Elderly
American Bar Association
1800 M Street, N.W.
Washington, DC 20036
(202) 331-2297

This arm of the ABA specializes in legal and policy issues affecting the elderly and can provide information on current and pending legislation.

National Senior Citizens Law Center
2025 M Street, N.W.
Washington, DC 20035

Advocating on behalf of elders, this professional organization sponsors conferences and workshops for attorneys wishing to specialize in elder affairs. A quarterly newsletter is available for a small fee.

National Institute on Aging Publications List
National Institute of Aging Information Center
Box 8057
Gaithersburg, MD 20898-8055

This publication, sent to you free of charge upon request, describes the many publications available free from this federal research agency that focuses on issues affecting the elderly.

Eldercare in the 90s
Friends and Relatives of the Institutionalized Aged
11 John Street, Suite 601
New York, NY 10038

This nonprofit advocacy group is dedicated to improving adult- and nursing-home conditions. This consumer's guide is done in a handy, loose-leaf notebook format and covers everything you need to know about care for the elderly. What questions to ask and what to look for, legal rights of the elderly, insurance, Medicaid, etc. To order ($25 plus $2.50 for postage and handling) just write to FRIA.

State Medicaid Offices

Most patients with Parkinson's disease will eventually need Medicaid, the federal insurance program to help them meet their financial and medical needs. The following is a list of Medicaid offices in every state.

Alabama
Dept. of Human Resources
64 N. Union St.
Montgomery, AL 36130
(205) 261-3190

Alaska
Div. of Public Assistance
Health & Social Services
P.O. Box H
Juneau, AK 99811

Arizona
Dept. of Economic Security
1717 W. Jefferson
Phoenix, AZ 85007
(602) 255-5678

Arkansas
Dept. of Human Services
1300 Donaghey Bldg.
Seventh & Main St.
Little Rock, AZ 72203
(501) 682-1001

California
Dept. of Social Services
744 P St.
Sacramento, CA 95814
(916) 445-2077

Colorado
Dept. of Social Services
717 17th St.
Denver, CO 80202
(303) 294-5800

Delaware
Div. of Economic Services
Health & Social Services
P.O. Box 906
New Castle, DE 19720
(302) 421-6734

Florida
Economic Services
Health & Rehabilitative Services
1311 Winwood Blvd.
Tallahasee, FL 32301
(904) 488-3271

Georgia
Family & Children Services
Dept. of Human Resources
878 Peachtree St. NE
Atlanta, GA 30309
(404) 894-6386

Hawaii
Public Welfare Div.
Dept. of Human Services
1390 Miller St.
Honolulu, HI 96813
(808) 548-5908

Idaho
Div. of Welfare
Dept. of Health & Welfare
450 W. State St.
Boise, ID 83720
(208) 334-5747

Illinois
Dept. of Public Aid
3163 Second St.
Springfield, IL 62762
(217) 782-6716

Indiana
Dept. of Public Welfare
100 N. Senate Ave., Rm. 701
Indianapolis, IN 46204
(317) 232-4705

Iowa
Bureau of Economic Assist.
Dept. of Human Services
Hoover State Office Bldg.
Des Moines, IA 50319
(515) 281-8629

Kansas
Income Maintenance
Dept. of Social and
Rehabilitative Services
6th Fl., State Office Bldg.
Topeka, KS 66612
(913) 296-3271

Louisiana
Office of Family Security
Health & Human Resources
P.O. Box 3776
Baton Rouge, LA 70621
(504) 342-3947

Maryland
Social Services Admin.
Dept. of Human Resources
300 W. Preston St.
Baltimore, MD 21201
(301) 263-5200

Michigan
Dept. of Social Services
300 S. Capitol Ave.
P.O. Box 30037
Lansing, MI 48909
(517) 373-3500

Mississippi
Dept. of Public Welfare
515 E. Amite St.
P.O. Box 352
Jackson, MS 39205
(601) 354-0341

Montana
Dept. of Social Services
111 Sanders St.
Helena, MT 59601
(406) 444-5622

Kentucky
Dept. of Social Insurance
Cabinet for Human Resources
275 E. Main St.
Frankfort, KY 40601
(502) 564-3703

Maine
Bureau of Income Maintenance
Dept. of Human Services
State House Station #11
Augusta, ME 04333
(207) 289-2415

Massachusetts
Dept. of Public Welfare
180 Tremont St.
Boston, MA 02111
(617) 727-6190

Minnesota
Assistance Payments, Policy and
  Operations Div.
444 Lafayette Rd.
St. Paul, MN 55101
(612) 296-6955

Missouri
Div. of Family Services
Dept. of Social Services
Broadway Bldg., Box 88
Jefferson City, MO 65013
(314) 751-4247

Nebraska
Dept. of Social Services
301 Centennial Mall S.
P.O. Box 95026
Lincoln, NE 68509
(402) 471-3121

Nevada
Div. of Welfare
Dept. of Human Resources
2527 N. Carfion St.
Carson City, NV 89710

New Jersey
Div. of Public Welfare
Dept. of Human Services
6 Quakerbridge Plaza
Trenton, NJ 08625
(609) 588-2401

New York
Dept. of Social Services
40 N. Pearl St.
Albany, NY 12243
(518) 474-9475

North Dakota
Dept. of Human Services
Judicial Wing, State Capitol
Bismarck, ND 58505
(710) 224-2310

Oklahoma
Dept. of Human Services
P.O. Box 25352
Oklahoma City, OK 73125
(405) 521-3646

Pennsylvania
Dept. of Public Welfare
333 Health & Welfare Bldg.
Harrisburg, PA 17120
(717) 787-2600

New Hampshire
Div. of Welfare
Dept. of Health and Welfare
Hazen Dr.
Concord, NH 03301
(603) 271-4321

New Mexico
Financial Assistance Bureau
Dept. of Human Services
P.O. Box 2348
Santa Fe, NM 87503
(505) 827-4429

North Carolina
Dept. of Human Resources
325 N. Salisbury St.
Raleigh, NC 27611
(919) 733-4534

Ohio
Dept. of Human Services
30 E. Broad St., 32nd Fl.
Columbus, OH 43266
(614) 466-6282

Oregon
Adult & Family Services Div.
Dept. of Human Resources
417 Public Service Bldg.
Salem, OR 97310
(503) 378-3680

Rhode Island
Social & Economic Services
Dept. of Social Services
600 New London Ave.
Cranston, RI 02920
(401) 464-2371

South Carolina
Dept. of Social Services
1535 Confederate Ave. Ext.
North Complex
Columbia, SC 29202
(803) 734-5760

Tennessee
Dept. of Human Services
111 Seventh Ave. N., 12th Fl.
Nashville, TN 37219
(615) 741-2341

Utah
Office of Assistance Payments
Dept. of Social Services
120 N. 200 W., 3rd Fl.
Salt Lake City, UT 84103
(801) 538-3970

Virginia
Dept. of Social Services
8007 Discovery Dr.
Richmond, VA 23288
(804) 281-9236

West Virginia
Dept. of Human Services
1900 Washington St. E.
Bldg. 6, Rm. 617-B
Charleston, WV 25305
(304) 348-2400

Wyoming
Public Assistance & Social Services
Health Dept.
Hathaway Building
Cheyenne, WY 82002
(307) 777-7564

South Dakota
Office of Program Mgt.
Dept. of Social Services
Kneip Bldg.
Pierre, SD 57501
(605) 773-3165

Texas
Dept. of Human Services
P.O. Box 2960
Austin, TX 78769
(512) 450-3030

Vermont
Dept. of Social Welfare
Agency of Human Services
103 S. Main St.
Waterbury, VT 05676
(802) 241-2853

Washington
Income Assistance Services
Dept. of Health Services
M/S OB-31C
Twelfth & Franklin
Olympia, WA 98504
(206) 753-3080

Wisconsin
Div. of Community Services
Dept. of Health & Social Services
One West Wilson St.
Box 7850
Madison, WI 53707
(608) 266-05854

District of Columbia
Income Maintenance Admn.
Dept. of Human Services
500 First St., N.W.
Rm. 9000
Washington, DC 20001
(202) 724-5506

Puerto Rico
Dept. of Social Services
P.O. Box 11398
Santurce, PR 00910
(809) 722-7400

Northern Mariana Islands
Dept. of Community Affairs
Office of the Governor
Salpan, CM 96950
(670) 322-9722

Virgin Islands
Dept. of Human Services
Barbel Plaza S.
St. Thomas, VI 00802
(809) 774-0930

Diseases That May Resemble Parkinson's Disease*

Benign Essential Tremor: A common condition that may appear in the elderly or the young and slowly progress over many years. The tremor is usually equal in both hands and increases when the hands are stretched out in front of the patient or when the hands are moving. The tremor may involve the head, but usually spares the legs. Patients with benign tremor have no other parkinsonian features, and there is usually a family history of tremor. In addition, parkinsonian tremor and benign tremor generally respond to different drugs. A small number of patients with benign essential tremor (less than 5 percent) may develop PD.

Shy-Drager Syndrome or Multisystem Atrophy: A condition in which the earliest and most severe symptoms are those of insufficiency of the autonomic nervous system: dizziness on standing, bladder difficulty, and impotence. These autonomic symptoms are followed by PD symptoms, such as rigidity, tremor, bradykinesia, postural instability, and gait difficulty. There is some question among neurologists as to whether the Shy-Drager Syndrome or Multisystem Atrophy is a form of PD or a separate disease.

Normal-Pressure Hydrocephalus: An uncommon condition that consists of difficulty in walking, mental changes, and urinary incontinence. This condition is caused by an enlargement of the fluid cavities in the brain which compress the parts of the brain that regulate walking, thinking, and voiding. Normal-pressure hydrocephalus differs from the more familiar hydrocephalus of childhood, which results from a blockage to the flow of

---

*Adapted from: *The Parkinson's Disease Handbook,* The American Parkinson's Disease Association, by A. N. Lieberman, M.D.; G. Gopinathan, M.D.; A. Neophytides, M.D., and M. Goldstein, Ph.D.

the spinal fluid. There is no known cause of this condition, which may be alleviated by a shunt (a tube placed in a ventricle which drains off the excess fluid).

Striatonigral Degeneration: A rare disorder in which patients become stiff and slow, and develop difficulty with balance and walking. Usually, patients do not have a tremor, but otherwise cannot be distinguished from patients with PD on the basis of a neurological exam. Patients with this condition, however, do not respond to anti-Parkinson medication, including levodopa. Most of the damage is in the striatum and not the substantia nigra. This is the reverse of the situation with PD. Only after death can this disorder be distinguished from PD. Magnetic resonance imaging (MRI) may sometimes disclose an increased deposition of iron in the putamen.

Pseudobulbar Palsy: A common disorder that occurs in patients with vascular disease of the brain (arteriosclerosis). Arteriosclerosis is especially likely to occur in patients with high blood pressure or diabetes. Patients who develop pseudobulbar palsy do so because they suffer a series of small strokes which are so mild that the patients are usually unaware of them. The ministrokes usually damage the part of the brain that controls balance and walking, the same area involved in PD. The two disorders may not be distinguished on the basis of a neurological examination alone. MRI may be especially useful in diagnosis. Patients with pseudobulbar palsy do not respond to anti-Parkinson drugs.

Progressive Supranuclear Palsy: An uncommon disorder in which patients develop paralysis of their eye movements, difficulty in speaking, rigidity, and senility. This disorder causes changes in the brain that are similar to those of PD, but are even more extensive. MRI may be useful in diagnosis.

Wilson's Disease: A rare, inherited metabolic disorder that appears in patients below the age of 40. Wilson's disease involves an inherited lack of a blood protein called ceruloplasmin, which carries the small amount of copper necessary for health. The lack of ceruloplasmin results in an excess accumulation of copper in the brain and in the liver, which eventually damages these two organs. Early diagnosis is important, as treatment is available to prevent further damage.

Hallervorden-Spatz Disease: A rare, inherited, progressive disease, Hallervorden-Spatz disease begins in late childhood. It is associated with the accumulation of excessive iron in certain parts of the brain. There is no treatment for this disease. MRI may be useful in diagnosis.

Olivopontocerebellar Degeneration: An uncommon disorder in which patients have difficulty with balance and walking, often called ataxia. The patients may have an action or postural tremor, but do not have rigidity or bradykinesia. The disorder results from a deterioration of certain structures in the nervous system, including the cerebellum, the pons (a part of the brainstem), and the olive (a part of the brainstem). This condition does not respond to anti-Parkinson drugs. MRI is helpful in diagnosis.

Huntington's Disease: A progressive hereditary disorder, usually beginning in early middle life, characterized by involuntary movements (dyskinesia, chorea) and changes in behavior, personality, and mood. The chorea, which resembles the dyskinesia experienced with an overdose of levodopa, may precede, occur simultaneously with, or follow the mental changes. The disease is caused by degeneration of nerve cells and actual tissue shrinkage in the basal ganglia and cortex of the brain. The disease, when fully developed, is easily distinguished from PD. However, the symptoms of a childhood form of Huntington's disease may resemble PD. Levodopa usually worsens the symptoms of Huntington's disease.

Dystonia: An inherited disease that begins in childhood and is progressive. The patients develop unusual postures of the head and neck, body, arms, and legs. This is called generalized dystonia (dystonia musculorum deformans). A variant of the disease, segmental dystonia, develops in adulthood and involves only one part of the body, e.g., the head and neck (torticollis or wryneck). Dystonia may rarely result from the use of certain drugs, such as phenothiazines. This type of dystonia will disappear when the offending drug is stopped.

Brain Tumors: Tumors of the brain that are close to the substantia nigra or the striatum may exert pressure on these structures, which often results in symptoms that resemble PD. A CT or MRI scan of the brain will exclude the possibility of a brain tumor as the cause of the parkinsonian symptoms.

Conditions Confused with PD

There are several relatively common neurological diseases that some patients confuse with Parkinson's disease, including two well-known conditions:

Multiple Sclerosis: A disease that begins in young adults and consists of a series of attacks on the myelin (fatty substance) of the white matter of the central nervous system. Why these attacks occur is unknown. They may result in a loss of vision, double vision, dizziness, loss of balance, paralysis, and bowel and bladder difficulty. There may be remissions during which the symptoms disappear. However, several attacks may damage the nervous system, resulting in permanent symptoms.

Amyotrophic Lateral Sclerosis (ALS, Lou Gehrig's Disease): Affecting more men than women, this disease begins in middle life. There is a progressive weakness and shrinkage (atrophy) of all the muscles of the body, including those that control speaking, eating, and breathing. There is no known cause or cure for this disease.

Glossary

Acetylcholine: a chemical which acts as a neurotransmitter. An imbalance between dopamine and acetylcholine results in some Parkinson's disease symptoms.

Action tremor: a tremor that increases when the hand is moving voluntarily.

Agonist: a drug which increases neurotransmitter activity by stimulating the dopamine receptors directly.

Akinesia: no movement.

Amantadine (Symmetrel): an anti-Parkinson drug (see Table 1).

Anticholinergics: anti-Parkinson drugs that block the action of acetylcholine, thereby rebalancing it in relation to dopamine and reducing rigidity and tremor; e.g., Artane, Cogentin (see Table 1).

Antihistamines: drugs that are often used to relieve cold or allergy symptoms (i.e., Benadryl) but may also be effective in reducing tremor.

Ataxia: loss of balance.

Athetosis: slow, involuntary movements of the hands and feet.

Atrophy: wasting, shrinkage.

Autonomic nervous system: that part of the nervous system that is responsible for automatic functions, such as the heartbeat, digestion, salivation.

Axon: the long, hairlike extension of a nerve cell that carries a message to the next nerve cell.

Basal ganglia: several large clusters of nerve cells deep in the brain below the cerebral hemispheres; crucial in coordinating motor commands. Include the striatum and the substantia nigra.

Bilateral: both sides of the body.

Biofeedback: a behavior modification in which patients are taught to partially control unconscious bodily functions, such as blood pressure or heart rate.

Blink rate: the number of times per minute that the eyelid automatically closes. A normal rate may be 10 to 30 per minute; for the parkinsonian it may be 0 to 5 per minute.

Blepharospasm: forced eyelid closure.

Blood-brain barrier: the protective membrane that separates circulating blood from brain cells.

Body scheme: the ability to identify body parts or to relate body parts to each other; the ability to sense one's position in space.

Bradykinesia: slowness of movement.

Bradyphrenia: slowness of thought processes.

Bromocriptine (Porlodel): a dopamine agonist and anti-Parkinson drug (see Table 1).

Bruxism: grinding of teeth and clenching of jaw muscles.

Buccinator: a muscle of the face and cheek.

Carbidopa: a drug that is used in combination with levodopa to treat PD. Carbidopa acts to prevent levodopa from being metabolized in the body, allowing more levodopa to reach the brain (see Table 1).

Central nervous system: the brain and the spinal cord.

Cerebellum: a large structure consisting of two halves (hemispheres) located in the lower part of the brain; responsible for the coordination of movement and balance.

Cerebrum: consists of two parts (lobes), left and right, which form the largest and most developed part of the brain; initiation and coordination of all voluntary movement take place within the cerebrum. The basal ganglia are located immediately below the cerebrum.

Chorea: rapid, jerky, dancelike movement of the body.

Cortex: the outer layer of the cerebrum, densely packed with nerve cells.

Dendrite: a threadlike extension from a nerve cell that serves as an antenna to receive messages from the axons of other nerve cells.

Delusions: a condition in which the patient has lost touch with reality and experiences hallucinations and misperceptions.

Deprenyl (Eldepryl, selegiline, Jumex): anti-Parkinson drug (see Table 1).

Dopa decarboxylase: an enzyme present in the body that converts levodopa to dopamine.

Dopa decarboxylase inhibitors: anti-Parkinson drugs that block the enzyme dopa decarboxylase.

Dopamine: a chemical substance, a neurotransmitter, found in the brain that regulates movement, balance, and walking. It is the substance that is lost in PD.

Dopaminergic: a chemical that works like, or has the same effect as, dopamine.

Drug holiday: a 3- to 14-day withdrawal of levodopa after long-term treatment when side effects of levodopa outweigh benefits; rarely done today because of the severe effects of drug withdrawal.

Dyskinesia: an involuntary movement including athetosis and chorea.

Dysphagia: difficulty in swallowing.

Dystonia: a slow movement or extended spasm in a group of muscles.

Edema: tissue swelling due to excessive fluid.

Enzyme: a substance that speeds up a specific chemical reaction but that is not itself consumed in the reaction.

Euphoria: a feeling of well-being or elation; may be drug-related.

Extensor (muscle): any muscle that causes the straightening of a limb or other part.

Extrapyramidal system: the system of nerve cells, nerve tracts and pathways that connects the cerebral cortex, basal ganglia, thalamus, cerebellum, reticular formation, and spinal neurons; it is concerned with the regulation of reflex movements such as balance and walking. The extrapyramidal system is damaged in Parkinson's disease.

Festination: short, shuffling steps; involuntary speeding up of the gait.

Flexor (muscle): any muscle that causes the bending of a limb or other body part.

Freezing: temporary, involuntary inability to move.

Ganglion: a cluster of nerve cells.

Gray matter: the darker-colored tissues of the central nervous system; in the brain, the gray matter includes the cerebral cortex, the thalamus, the basal ganglia, and the outer layers of the cerebellum.

Hormone: a substance secreted by a gland that is transported in the bloodstream to various organs in order to regulate or modify bodily functions.

Incontinence: involuntary voiding of the bladder or bowel.

Levodopa: the single most effective anti-Parkinson drug which is changed into dopamine in the brain usually combined with carbidopa (a dopa decarboxylase inhibitor) as Sinemet (see Table 1).

Lewy body: a pink-staining sphere, found in the bodies of dying cells, that is considered to be a marker for Parkinson's disease.

Micrographia: a change in handwriting with the script becoming smaller and more cramped.

Monoamine oxidase (MAO): an enzyme that breaks down dopamine.

There are two types of MAO: "A" and "B." In Parkinson's disease, it is beneficial to block the activity of MAO B.

MPTP: a chemical produced during an attempt to make a synthetic narcotic. MPTP destroys the cells of the substantia nigra cells and produces a disease that mimics Parkinson's disease.

Myoclonus: jerking, involuntary movements of the arms and legs. May occur normally during sleep.

Neuron: a cell specialized to conduct and generate electrical impulses and to carry information from one part of the brain to another.

Neurotransmitters: chemical substances that carry impulses from one nerve cell to another; found in the space (synapse) that separates the transmitting neuron's terminal (axon) from the receiving neuron's terminal (dendrite).

Nigral: of or referring to the substantia nigra.

Norepinephrine: a neurotransmitter found mainly in areas of the brain that are involved in governing autonomic nervous system activity, especially blood pressure and heart rate.

On-off phenomena: abrupt changes in performance during the day caused by the taking effect or wearing off of anti-Parkinson drugs.

Orthostatic hypotension: a large decrease in blood pressure upon standing; may result in fainting. Orthostatic hypertension may occur spontaneously in PD or may be related to certain drugs.

Palsy: paralysis of a muscle or group of muscles.

Pergolide (Permax): an anti-Parkinson drug (see Table 1).

Peristalsis: wavelike contractions that move food through the digestive tract.

Pyramidal pathway: a collection of nerve tracts that travel from the cerebral cortex through the pyramid of the medulla oblongata in the brainstem to the spinal cord. Within the pyramid of the medulla, fibers cross from one side of the brain to the opposite side of the spinal cord; the pyramidal pathway is intact in Parkinson's disease.

Range of motion: the extent that a joint will move from full extension to full flexion.

Resting tremor: a tremor of a limb that increases when the limb is at rest.

Rigidity: increased resistance to the passive movement of a limb.

Sialorrhea: drooling.

Sinemet: an anti-Parkinson drug (see Table 1).

Spasm: a condition in which a muscle or group of muscles involuntarily contract.

Striatum: part of the basal ganglia, it is a large cluster of nerve cells, consisting of the caudate nucleus and the putamen, that controls movement, balance, and walking; the neurons of the striatum require dopamine to function.

Substantia nigra: a small area of the brain containing a cluster of black-pigmented nerve cells that produce dopamine which is then transmitted to the striatum.

Sustention (postural) tremor: a tremor of a limb that increases when the limb is stretched.

Synapse: a tiny gap between the ends of nerve fibers across which nerve impulses pass from one neuron to another; at the synapse, an impulse causes the release of a neurotransmitter, which diffuses across the gap and triggers an electrical impulse in the next neuron.

Tremor: a rhythmical shaking of a limb, head, mouth, tongue, or other part of the body.

Tyrosine: the amino acid from which dopamine is made.

White matter: nerve tissue that is paler in color than gray matter because it contains nerve fibers with large amounts of insulating material (myelin). The white matter does not contain nerve cells. In the brain, the white matter lies within the gray layer of the cerebral cortex.

INDEX

About the Authors

ABRAHAM N. LIEBERMAN, M.D., is a board-certified neurologist who is Chief of Movement Disorders at the Barrow Neurological Institute in Phoenix, Arizona, and Chairman of the Medical Advisory Board of the American Parkinson's Disease Association (APDA). He had been Professor of Neurology at New York University Medical Center. He has been the recipient of numerous research grants and awards used to study various aspects of Parkinson's disease.

FRANK L. WILLIAMS is the Executive Director of the APDA, a national organization that educates people about Parkinson's disease, supports those afflicted with the disease and raises funds to continue research. He is the founder of APDA's Operation Outreach, a program serving the nation's Parkinson's community through symposia and seminars, Information and Referral Centers, chapters and support groups. He lives in Staten Island, New York, with his wife and two sons.

SUSAN IMKE, R.N., M.S., is a nurse practitioner certified in gerontology and family health care by the American Nurses Association. She holds a master's degree in community health education and currently practices in the Division of Neurology at the Barrow Neurological Institute in Phoenix. She also serves as coordinator of the APDA's Information and Referral Center in Central Arizona, and is active in the American Association of Neuroscience Nursing, and the American Academy of Nurse Practitioners.

ELLEN MOSCINSKI, L.C.S.W., M.S.W., is Director of Social Work at Maine Medical Center in Portland. She completed her graduate work in health-care social work at San Diego State University, where she was also an adjunct professor. She has served as an expert examiner for the state of California's Board of Behavioral Sciences, and was the coordinator of the APDA Information and Referral Center in San Diego. She is the past president of both the San Diego Chapter of the National Association of Social Workers' Health Council, and the Southern California Chapter of the Society of Hospital Social Work Directors.

PAULA BENOIST FALWELL, P.T., is a physical therapist who works extensively with Parkinson's disease patients. She is a contributing author of the APDA handbook for physical therapists entitled *Coping with Parkinson's Disease*. She is the founder of the Parkinson's Disease Video Library in Washington, D.C., and has produced a two-part home-exercise video called *Rhythm and Moves*, designed to address the problems encountered by persons with Parkinson's disease. She is currently in private practice in Washington, D.C.

HARLEY GORDON, ESQ., is an attorney who lectures extensively on the effects of Parkinson's disease on a family's finances. He is a founding member and former director of The National Academy of Elder Law Attorneys. He is the author of *How to Protect Your Life Savings from Catastrophic Illness and Nursing Homes*. An active speaker who has appeared on numerous nationally broadcast television news and talk shows, he was featured in PBS's *Frontline:* "Who Pays for Mom and Dad?" He lives and practices in Boston, Massachusetts.

SUZANNE LEVERT is a writer and editor who specializes in health-related subjects. She is the author of *If It Runs in the Family: Hypertension, Teens Face to Face with Chronic Illness*, and *AIDS: In Search of a Killer*. She lives in Cambridge, Massachusetts.